CHILDBEARING AMONG HISPANICS IN THE UNITED STATES

Recent Titles in
Bibliographies and Indexes in Women's Studies

Women in China: A Selected and Annotated Bibliography
Karen T. Wei

Women Writers of Spain: An Annotated Bio-Bibliographical Guide
Carolyn L. Galerstein and Kathleen McNerney, editors

The Equal Rights Amendment: An Annotated Bibliography of the Issues,
1976-1985
Renee Feinberg, compiler

Women Writers of Spanish America: A Bio-Bibliographical Guide
Diane E. Marting, editor

CHILDBEARING AMONG HISPANICS IN THE UNITED STATES

An Annotated Bibliography

Compiled by **KATHERINE F. DARABI**

With assistance from: Marysol Asencio, Dana Brodsky, Zenobia Ferguson, Anne Gardner, Jay Kantor, Jodi Katz, Amy Koff, Leandra Lederman, Joyce Sackey *of the Center for Population and Family Health, Faculty of Medicine, Columbia University*

Bibliographies and Indexes in Women's Studies, Number 4

GREENWOOD PRESS
New York • Westport, Connecticut • London

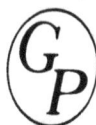

Library of Congress Cataloging-in-Publication Data

Darabi, Katherine F.
  Childbearing among Hispanics in the United
States.

  (Bibliographies and indexes in women's studies,
ISSN 0742-6941 ; no. 4)
  Includes indexes.
  1. Fertility, Human—United States—Bibliography.
2. Birth control—United States—Bibliography.
3. Hispanic Americans—Bibliography. 4. Pregnancy,
Adolescent—United States—Bibliography. 5. Hispanic-
American youth—Bibliography. I. Title. II. Series
Z7164.D3D27 1987   016.3046'32'08968073   86-33716
[HB915]
ISBN 0-313-25617-9 (lib. bdg. : alk. paper)

This research was supported by the Carnegie Corporation.
The opinions expressed herein are those of the authors and do not
necessarily reflect the view of the Carnegie Corporation.

Library of Congress Catalog Card Number: 86-33716
ISBN: 0-313-25617-9
ISSN: 0742-6941

First published in 1987

Greenwood Press, Inc.
88 Post Road West, Westport, Connecticut 06881

Printed in the United States of America

∞

The paper used in this book complies with the
Permanent Paper Standard issued by the National
Information Standards Organization (Z39.48-1984).

10 9 8 7 6 5 4 3 2 1

Contents

Preface   vii

Introduction   xi

Part One: Fertility Determinants

1. General Fertility Determinants   1

2. Sex-Related Attitudes and Knowledge   22

3. Marriage and Household Structure   54

4. Sexual Activity   68

Part Two: Pregnancy and Fertility

1. Pregnancy and Prenatal Care   70

2. Abortion   75

3. Fertility   83

Part Three: Fertility Regulation

1. Family Planning Services and Clients   98

2. Contraceptive Use: Reversible Methods   113

3. Sterilization   125

Part Four: Consequences of Childbearing

1. Programs and Consequences for Adolescent
    Parents   130

2. Fertility Consequences for Adults   142

Part Five: General Topics

    1.   Overviews of Hispanics   147

    2.   Hispanic Males   153

Author Index   159

Subject Index   165

Preface

This comprehensive bibliography contains abstracts of 364 articles concerning the fertility-related attitudes and behavior of Hispanics in the United States. The bibliography is part of a Carnegie Corporation-sponsored research project designed to improve our knowledge of these topics in relation to Hispanic adolescents. It is the product of two years of work reviewing approximately 5,000 bibliographic citations from health and social science data bases, files of government publications, references in published articles, tables of contents of journals, and library card catalogues and indices.

Many individuals assisted in the preparation of this bibliography. Special thanks go to Carole Oshinsky, Jan Watterworth, and Susan Pasquariella for their contributions and advice and assistance securing materials and inputting relevant citations into the POPLINE system; to Norman Weatherby for computer programming assistance in the retrieval and downloading of citations for the bibliography; and to the bibliographic specialists and abstractors from POPLINE, MEDLINE, Psych INFO, Health Planning, SSCI, SOCA, NIMH, and ERIC who supplied many important references and abstracts.

The bibliography surveys articles written during the past fifteen years on the subject of Hispanics in the continental United States, and their attitudes or behavior concerning marital status, sexual activity, pregnancy, abortion, childbearing, and contraceptive use. Clinical medical articles were excluded, and only selected, especially pertinent dissertations were accepted. Relevant articles were identified through manual searches and by computerized searches of the POPLINE, MEDLINE, Health Planning, Psych INFO, SSCI, SOCA, NIMH, and ERIC data bases.

Several features of the bibliography enhance its usefulness. Because of widespread interest in adolescent pregnancy and childbearing as separate topics, each article which contains data on adolescents or a discussion of teenage pregnancy is marked with an asterisk before the autnor's name. For example:

14. *Beckman LJ. The relationship between sex roles, fertility, and family size preferences. **Psychology of Women Quarterly.** 1979 Fall;4(1):43-6.

Another substantive area of particular interest is country of origin. Researchers in Florida, for example, may be particularly interested in articles concerned with Cubans in the United States, while scholars in New York may be most interested in studies of Puerto Ricans or Dominicans. Data or discussions of groups from particular countries of origin are designated by bold face within each abstract as follows:

30. Linn MW ; Gurel L ; Carmichael J ; Weed P. Cultural comparisons of mothers with large and small families. **Journal of Bio-social Science.** 1976;8:293-302.

Contraceptive knowledge and behavior of mothers of large (five or more children) and small (under three children) families in four subcultures were compared with white Protestants. Four hundred and forty-nine mothers aged 30 to 45 years were studied from black, **Cuban,** Indian, **Mexican,** and white groups. With social class, knowledge of birth control, and degree of religiosity held constant, the best predictors of family size were the mother's desired family size (expressed as desired minus actual children), age at childbirth, and age at marriage. Data suggest that family size is not purely a function of birth control knowledge, but related to early marriage and pregnancy, and in keeping with attitudes about an ideal family size. In general, factors related to size were stronger in the white group than in the other groups. In a few instances certain cultures were not consistent with others in overall trends. Any intervention program needs to be aware of differences in motivation that arise from cultural influence.

There are several ways to find abstracts on particular topics of interest. The bibliography is organized into subject headings under the broad categories of "Fertility Determinants," "Pregnancy and Fertility," "Fertility Regulation," "Consequences of Childbearing," and "General Topics." Individual chapters within these categories are outlined in the contents. Further detail on the topics covered in each area is in the introductory page for each section. These introductory sections summarize important findings on each of the chapter topics and point out areas of needed research. In addition, specific variables or measures included in articles within each chapter are summarized and printed in boldface type in the introduction. For example, the introduction to the chapter on "Fertility Determinants" mentions that "measures of acculturation or assimilation have included **pre- and post-migration comparisons, legal status, generation, and English language proficiency.**"

A detailed subject index and an author and co-author index are included at the end of the bibliography. These indexes refer to abstracts by the numbers preceding each bibliographic

entry.   For   example,   articles   on income as a determinant   of
fertility   can be found in eight abstracts in the   bibliography.
These abstracts are listed under the entry in the subject   index
as follows:

    Fertility, general determinants of:
        income, 2-3, 11-12, 17-18, 39, 215.

Introduction

Hispanics represent the fastest growing minority group in the United States. This is due not only to immigration but also to the well-publicized fact that Hispanic adults, as a group, have a higher fertility rate than adults in other ethnic groups in the United States.

Although there is considerable interest in the demography of Hispanics in the United States, comprehensive information on this topic is difficult to obtain because it appears in widely disparate sources. Relevant articles on Hispanic fertility can be found in numerous publications that deal with subjects as varied as psychology, education, sociology, minority studies, demography, and mental and public health, as well as in published and unpublished documents from conferences, doctoral work, and federal agencies. Thus, numerous bibliographic searches on different data bases and through large numbers of irrelevant or duplicated citations are required in order to find useful material. This comprehensive bibliography was compiled in order to assist researchers, students, program administrators, policy makers, and others interested in Hispanic fertility and any related topics, obtain any available information more easily and quickly.

The sections of the bibliography are organized following the general schema of a model of the determinants and consequences of fertility, followed by a section of special topics. From the data presented, it can be concluded that numerous studies have demonstrated the existence of differences in birth rates between Hispanic and non-Hispanic women, and among some of the various groups of Hispanic origin, but that the causes and consequences of these differences are imperfectly understood. Particularly lacking are data concerning the role of cultural beliefs and practices upon sexuality, pregnancy, and fertility. This is significant because it means many of the commonly espoused theories concerning the influence of machismo, familism, religiosity, and authoritarian family values on these behaviors actually have not been tested empirically.

Because persons of Mexican origin represent over 60% of all Hispanics in the United States, the bulk of research, and therefore the bulk of studies abstracted in this bibliography, focus upon Chicanos. This is misleading since the few available comparative studies demonstrate marked differences in fertility among the various groups of Hispanic origin. Much less is known about the fertility-related attitudes and behavior of some of the less populous Hispanic groups, particularly those which are not identified separately in the United States Census. An agenda for future research should include not only comparisons of sexual activity, fertility, and contraceptive use among groups of Hispanic origin within the continental United States, but also cross-cultural studies which permit contrasts of Hispanic women in their countries of origin and in the United States.

Cross-cultural studies would also be useful for a better understanding of adolescent childbearing in Hispanic communities in the United States. The goal of such research should be to shed light upon the process of acculturation and the ways in which sex-related attitudes and norms are transmitted to adolescents in their countries of origin and in the continental United States.

Hispanic males have been ignored in fertility-related research much as they have been left out of this type of research on non-Hispanic populations. The importance of studies on the attitudes and behavior of Hispanic adolescent males and adult males is obvious given the preponderance of theories concerning their pro-natalist and traditional sex role attitudes.

Attention to the Hispanic family unit and the interrelationships among parents, children, and extended family members would be another important contribution to the field. Little is known about such important topics as patterns of communication about sex and the formation of aspirations for marriage, childbearing, and careers. Another neglected topic concerns consensual marital unions among Hispanics. Although we know that such unions are common among some groups of Hispanic origin, the conventional survey questions regarding civil marriage do not permit an examination of these alternative union patterns. There is a need for good research which examines the fertility effects of such living situations as consensual unions, extended families, and single parent households.

Finally, any discussion of needed research on Hispanic fertility must emphasize the importance of oversampling* Hispanic respondents and of carefully identifying them in sociological studies and on clinic utilization forms, not only by including self-identification questions with detailed lists of groups of Hispanic origin, but also measures of ancestry and place of birth. It is only by accumulating repeated measures with consistent definitions of Hispanic ethnicity and acculturation that some of the gaps in our knowledge of the fertility-related attitudes and behavior of Hispanics in the United States can be overcome.

*Since persons of Hispanic origin constitute only about seven percent of the United States population, even large survey samples often include few Hispanic respondents. In order to examine the characteristics of Hispanics, it is often necessary to include more than seven percent of them in a study by "oversampling."

CHILDBEARING AMONG HISPANICS IN THE UNITED STATES

PART ONE
FERTILITY DETERMINANTS
1. General Fertility Determinants

For many years demographers have observed that Mexicans in the United States have higher birth rates and larger families than non-Hispanic adults. Research to explain these differences in both current and cumulative fertility has built upon earlier theories of the determinants of black/white differentials. In general terms sociologists have been interested in the extent to which members of minority groups have higher or lower fertility because of what has been termed structural or compositional differences (such as age, socioeconomic status, years of schooling or rural residence) and to what extent other culturally determined differences remain once these background characteristics are held constant. Goldscheider and Uhlenberg (1969) refined earlier theories on this topic by postulating that, while socioeconomic variables are important determinants of fertility, minority status exerts its own independent effect. They explained the lower fertility of some U.S. minority groups by postulating that "membership in, and identification with a minority group which does not have a normative system encouraging large families, and which does not prohibit or discourage the use of efficient methods of contraception, depresses fertility below majority levels."

Specific studies of Mexican American and non-Hispanic fertility have tested the inverse of this theory: that is, whether membership in a minority group which has pronatalist norms raises fertility above majority levels net of socioeconomic background characteristics of the group members. Research on this topic has generally supported the Goldscheider and Uhlenberg hypothesis, and suggests that cultural or minority group membership factors interact with socioeconomic characteristics.

Among the structural or compositional variables in this section which have been related to Mexican American fertility are employment, income, education, marital status, and urban residence. Measures of acculturation or assimilation have included pre- and post-migration comparisons, legal status, generation, and English language proficiency.

2   General Fertility Determinants

Those few studies which have examined fertility determinants among Hispanic origin groups other than Mexicans (notably
Puerto Ricans), suggest that for them the effects of migration
and assimilation may be very different. Hispanic adolescents
represent another understudied group who are likely to behave
very differently from Hispanic adults because of cohort effects
and the differing effects of marital status, education and
family size desires on adolescent and adult fertility.

1. *Abrahamse AF ; Morrison PA ; Waite LJ. How family characteristics deter early unwed parenthood. Paper presented at the
Annual Population Association of America Meeting, Boston, Massachusetts. March 28-30, 1985. (Unpublished) 31 p.

This paper examines the risk of unwed motherhood during mid-
adolescence and certain factors (including parental influences)
which suppress that risk. The research is based on data from a
large, nationally representative sample of high school sophomores, of which a small fraction were mothers who were not
married in their senior year. Sharp differences were found in
the risk of unwed parenthood when the adolescent population is
stratified by a few background variables. Strong and consistent
relationships between risk of parenthood and: 1) three racial
groups--blacks, Hispanics, and all other races (consisting
mostly of whites); 2) socioeconomic status; 3) the young
woman's academic ability; and 4) being in a female-headed family
were found. After controls for each of the latter three independent variables, the risk of unwed parenthood was lowest for
whites, mid-level for Hispanics, and highest for blacks.

2. Bean FD. Components of income and expected family size among
Mexican Americans. In: Tien HY and Bean FD, eds. **Comparative
family and fertility research.** Leiden EJ Brill. 1974. p. 174-87.
(International studies in sociology and social anthropology, Vol
17).

Examines fertility differentials by income among **Mexican** Americans, considering several hypotheses relevant to the interrela-
tionship between income and fertility. The currently emerging
"economic theory of family formation" stresses the importance of
potential and actual financial resources for fertility decisions. To accommodate this interpretation of fertility behavior, it is desirable to decompose the income variable as a
preliminary strategy for measuring income as delineated by the
economic theory. The proposed decomposition would reflect
"absolute" socioeconomic status (essentially a statement of
"expected" income values reflective of "social status" income);
and "relative" socioeconomic status (determined by the difference between actual and expected social status income). The
relations between these income components and fertility, and
their interactions with other variables are examined, and the
results are discussed in terms of their implications for the
economic theory of family formation.

3. Bean FD. Social status components of income and fertility
differences among Mexican Americans. Austin, Texas, University
of Texas, Texas Population Research Center. 1972. 24 p.

This paper examines fertility differentials by income among
Mexican Americans. Alternative hypotheses relevant to the
income/fertility relation are considered. The author proposes a

decomposition of the income variable as a preliminary strategy to dealing with the problem of measuring income posed by the economic theory. The analysis of the relations between social income and relative income and fertility is based on data from the 1969 Austin Family Survey, which consisted of a sample of 348 Mexican American couples, married three years or more. The dependent variable in the analysis is expected family size rather than current family size. The two components of income were derived from husband's current income. The plan of analysis is to examine fertility differentials by the two measures of income, and then to observe these as affected by other variables which may be thought to influence the income/fertility relationship. The relations between the income components and fertility, as well as their interactions with other variables are examined, and the results are discussed in terms of their implications for the economic theory of family formation.

4. Bean FD ; Cullen RM ; Stephen EH ; Swicegood CG. Generational differences in fertility among Mexican Americans: implications for assessing the effects of immigration. **Social Science Quarterly**. 1984 Jun;65(2):573-82.

The impact of generational differences on fertility among **Mexican** Americans is analyzed. The authors then examine the effects of generation on both current and cumulative fertility for a sample disaggregated by age group. The 1970 Public Use Sample data are used for this research because they enable the employment of a three-generational breakdown of the Mexican origin population. The basic purpose of the research is to examine fertility differentials between other whites and generational groups within the Mexican American population. It is found that there is a clear tendency toward fertility reduction the longer the familial exposure to life in the United States. This even involves convergence to levels of non-Hispanic white women's current fertility in the case of many third and later-generation women. The effects of international migration and of early, possibly subculturally related, patterns of childbearing on Mexican origin fertility operate in such a way to make this pattern less detectable, thus helping to explain the negative and conflicting results of earlier studies. Overall, however, the pattern of results is consistent with the notion that both subcultural and assimilationist forces influence the fertility behavior of Mexican Americans.

5. Bean FD ; Frisbie WP. Some issues in the demographic study of racial and ethnic populations. In: Bean FD and Frisbie WP, eds. **The demography of racial and ethnic groups**. New York, Academic Press. 1978. p. 1-14.

Research into demographic variation by race, ethnicity, or minority group status has led to several different ways of classifying the determinants of this behavior. The approach which searches for determinants of demographic variation in the history and cultural traditions of different subpopulations is referred to as the cultural approach. By contrast, the structural approach seeks an explanation in the extent to which subpopulations have obtained access to and have been assimilated into the economic and political structures of the larger society. The characteristics or assimilationist hypothesis attributes fertility differentials to dissimilarities between groups in regard to various social, demographic, and economic characteristics. Still another hypothesis comes from the finding that the fertility of high socioeconomic status members of some groups is lower than that of their majority counterparts. Goldscheider and Uhlenberg explain this result in terms of the insecurity that accompanies minority group status. Whatever the adequacy of their explanation, the observed pattern suggests the possibility that group membership and social and economic characteristics interact in their effects on fertility.

6.   Bean FD ; Marcum JP. Differential fertility and the minority group status hypothesis: an assessment and review. In: Bean FD and Frisbie WP, eds. **The demography of racial and ethnic groups.** New York City, Academic Press. 1978. p. 189-211.

It has long been recognized that fertility differentials existed among various racial and ethnic groups in the United States. Of groups charted, only **Cubans** and Japanese Americans have a lower average fertility than native born, urban whites; all other groups including **Mexicans** and **Puerto Ricans** exceed the majority fertility.   The social characteristics hypothesis regarding the differentials between minority and majority groups sees the differences tied to the distribution of socioeconomic factors. The minority group status hypothesis posits the view that minority status operates as an independent factor influencing fertility.   Various studies which have tested these two hypotheses of differential minority fertility are cited.   Problems with this type of research are: 1) the definition of a minority group; 2) methodology; and 3) the lack of clarity as to what evidence would prove either theory. The effects of generations and place of residence must also be considered.

7.   Bean FD ; Swicegood CG. Generation, female education and Mexican American fertility. **Social Science Quarterly.** 1982 Mar; 63(1):131-44.

Based upon data for a **Mexican** American and other white sample drawn from the 1976 Survey of Income and Education, it was found that current and cumulative Mexican American fertility decrease both with length of exposure to the receiving society (measured by generation) and with rising socioeconomic status (measured by female education).   Moreover, most Mexican American women of later-generation and greater education manifest even lower cumulative fertility than would be expected considering indicators of these variables separately.   Differences in cumulative and current fertility between Mexican American and other white women are reduced substantially, but not eliminated when female education is held constant; the differences are not much further affected when the other control variables are introduced. Other things being equal, differences in cumulative fertility between later-generation Mexican Americans and other whites tend to vary curvilinearly with female education, women of intermediate educational attainment showing the least fertility difference.   The pattern of results is interpreted as suggesting a modified theory of minority group status effects on fertility.

8.   Bean FD ; Swicegood CG. **Mexican American fertility patterns.** Austin, Texas, University of Texas Press. 1985. 178 p.

The primary purpose of the research reported in this monograph has been to investigate fertility patterns among **Mexican** Americans.   The authors have focused on the possibility that residence in the United States, a country with lower fertility than Mexico, might serve to influence the fertility behavior of

Mexican immigrant women and their descendants.   They have also
emphasized the theoretical and empirical utility of invoking the
idea of opportunity costs in developing explanations of minority
fertility patterns.   The opportunity costs framework also contributes substantially to understanding the forces lying behind
reduced fertility among certain categories of Mexican American
women.   For example, in general, the later-generational women
with higher educations are the ones most likely to show low
levels of childbearing. Furthermore, this tendency is most evident under the circumstance where the external structure of
socioeconomic opportunities available to these women is greatest.   Neither the subcultural, the social characteristics, or
the minority group status approaches provide a basis for explaining these patterns.

9.   Bean FD ; Swicegood CG ; Linsley TF. Patterns of fertility
variation among Mexican immigrants to the United States. Austin,
Texas, University of Texas, Texas Population Research Center.
1981. 65 p. (Texas Population Research Center Paper No. 2.016).

This paper tests the hypothesis that members of the population
of Mexican descent (Mexican Americans) decrease their fertility
depending upon the length of time spent in the United States,
and that this tendency is more pronounced among couples of
higher socioeconomic status.   Data come from the 1970 U.S.
Public Use Samples and the 1976 Survey of Income and Education.
In general, the findings are consistent with the idea that
Mexican American fertility is similar to majority fertility
under conditions of greater acculturation and structural assimilation. Mexican American fertility is observed to decrease both
with length of exposure to the receiving society (measured by
generation) and with rising socioeconomic status (measured by
female education).   The results also suggest that processes of
acculturation and structural assimilation jointly influence the
cumulative fertility of Mexican American women.   Mexican American women of greater education and later-generation manifest
even lower fertility than would be expected considering indicators of these variables separately.

10.   *Bean FD ; Swicegood CG ; Marcum JP. Minority group status
and patterns of Mexican American and black fertility. Austin,
Texas, University of Texas, Texas Population Research Center.
1983. 36 p. (Texas Population Research Center Paper No. 5.018).

This study investigates the relationship between female education and fertility among Mexican Americans and blacks in the
United States.   Using 1970 U.S. Census Public Use Sample data
the authors found that for Mexican American women, the most
negative educational/fertility relationships occur among younger
women, who would be expected to have enjoyed greater access to
resources than older women.   For blacks, the opposite pattern
emerges in which the most negative relationships occur among
older black women who would be expected to have experienced less
access.   It is concluded that the forces outlined by the minority group status hypothesis provide a basis for interpreting
more steeply declining fertility with rising education among
blacks, but that the forces behind the different opportunity
costs perspective provide a better basis for interpreting   this
relationship among Mexican Americans.

11.   Bean FD ; Swicegood CG ; Marcum JP. Social context and the
relationship between female education and Mexican American fer-

tility. Paper presented at the 52nd Annual Meeting of the Population Association of America, Pittsburgh, Pennsylvania. April
14-16, 1983. (Unpublished) 6 p.

Five tables concerned with the social context and the relationship between female education and **Mexican** American fertility
present the following: descriptive statistics for variables
used in the analysis of the fertility of ever married Mexican
American women by cohort, 1970; regressions of number of children ever born on independent variables; four cohorts of ever
married Mexican American women, 1970; regressions of number of
children less than six on independent variables; four cohorts of
ever married black women, 1970. The independent variables used
were: wife's education; generation one or generation two; Spanish; neighborhood fertility; age; rural/urban residence; marital
disruption; labor force participation; and family income.   It
was hypothesized that fertility would vary with social distance
i.e., that the lower the percent Spanish in the neighborhood the
more negative the effects of education on fertility and the
younger the age cohort.

12. Bean FD ; Wood CH. Ethnic variations in the relationship
between income and fertility. **Demography.** 1974 Nov;11(4):629-40.

The effects of husband's potential and relative income on completed fertility, as well as their effects on certain parity
progression probabilities, are examined within samples of Anglos, blacks and **Mexican** Americans. Relationships are estimated
using data from the one percent 1960 and 1970 United States
Public Use Samples. The results reveal different patterns of
relationship by ethnicity between the measures of income and the
measures of fertility. The effects on completed fertility of
the income measures are positive for Anglos and negative for
blacks, while in the case of Mexican Americans the effect of
potential income is negative and that of relative income is
positive.   Income effects on the parity progression probabilities are similar in pattern to those from the analyses using
completed fertility, although somewhat different patterns tend
to appear at different birth orders, especially among Anglos.

13. *Becerra RM ; De Anda D. Pregnancy and motherhood among
Mexican American adolescents. **Health and Social Work.** 1984
Spring;9(2):106-23.

The influence of acculturation among **Mexican** American adolescents was examined in reference to attitudes toward pregnancy
and motherhood, contraceptive and reproductive knowledge, and
the role of family and peers both as behavioral models and as
support networks.   Data were collected by administering questionnaires to 122 adolescent participants of the Los Angeles
County Supplementary Food Program for Women, Infants, and
Children.   Each of two cohorts was subdivided into the three
categories of less acculturated Mexican Americans, more acculturated Mexican Americans, and white non-Hispanics.   The less
acculturated Mexican Americans were more likely than other
groups to follow the Mexican tradition of marrying if a pregnancy occurred.   Less acculturated Mexican Americans were more
likely to discontinue their schooling when they became pregnant
than other adolescents. The more acculturated Mexican Americans
were more knowledgeable about reproduction than other subgroups,
but they were less likely to use contraceptives than the other
groups.   They were also more likely to reject parental guide-

lines and to have a higher proportion of unplanned pregnancies than the other groups.

14. *Beckman LJ. The relationship between sex roles, fertility, and family size preferences. **Psychology of Women Quarterly**. 1979 Fall;4(1):43-6.

Interview data collected from a sample of 583 currently married women living in Los Angeles County in California were used to assess the impact of sex role attitudes and behavior on fertility and the impact of fertility on sex role attitudes and behavior. Sixty-one percent of the respondents were Anglos, 23% were Hispanic, and nine percent were black. Correlation analysis revealed that: 1) the relationship between sex roles and fertility was not strong; 2) the relationship was strongest among blacks and weakest among Hispanics; 3) sex role attitudes for blacks were more closely related to fertility than sex role behavior within the family; and 4) past and present employment was closely related to fertility for all three groups. Path analysis revealed that Anglo women with more traditional attitudes wanted more children than those with non-traditional attitudes, but that women who performed most of the housework in their families desired fewer children than those women who shared housework with their husbands.

15. Cooney RS ; Rogler LH ; Schroder E. Puerto Rican fertility: an examination of social characteristics, assimilation, and minority status variables. **Social Forces**. 1981 Jun;58(4):1094-113.

The Goldscheider/Uhlenberg theory of minority group fertility was examined by making a direct assessment of the importance of assimilation and minority status variables on **Puerto Rican** fertility behavior before and after controlling for social characteristics. The study population consisted of 200 currently married Puerto Rican women participating in a larger study of continuity and change in the Puerto Rican family. The following were the major study findings: 1) assimilation was of limited usefulness in studying the fertility behavior of either the older or younger generation of Puerto Rican wives studied, for it failed to increase understanding of Puerto Rican fertility behavior beyond what is known to be the effect of social characteristics; and 2) minority status insecurity had a substantial direct effect on the fertility of the younger generation. Goldscheider and Uhlenberg's contention that striving for primary group acceptance is associated with insecurities that manifest themselves in lowered fertility was supported by the significance of unfulfilled desire for non-Puerto Rican friends, after controlling for social characteristics.

16. Curry JP ; Scriven GD. The relationship between apartment living and fertility for blacks, Mexican Americans, and other Americans in Racine, Wisconsin. **Demography**. 1978 Nov;15(4):477-85.

Recently published data from a sample of Bogota, Columbia public housing residents show that apartment dwellers, but not house dwellers, reduced their fertility in a tight housing market. The authors propose that the utility cost theory of fertility accounts for this finding, and using this theory, they predict that: apartment residents will not decrease their fertility in an open housing market; and higher fertility will be associated with larger dwellings. Longitudinal data from a sample of midwest urban blacks, **Mexican** Americans, and other Americans support both predictions. The substantive implications are discussed. There is no strong evidence to show that a government's desire to reduce fertility through a controlled housing program would succeed. The possible adverse effects of density and other unforeseen consequences would seem to advise against such a policy. On the other hand, a well considered housing policy may be a realistic alternative to other methods of fertility control where the society is faced with both housing shortages and a population problem.

17. Falasco D ; Heer DM. Economic and fertility differences between legal and undocumented migrant Mexican families: possible effects of immigration policy changes. **Social Science Quarterly**. 1984 Jun;65(2):495-504.

Utilizing cross-sectional data comparing the current socioeconomic characteristics and fertility of 500 legal and undocumented **Mexican** migrants currently in Los Angeles County, a model is developed to determine how legal status might affect fertility within the context of the economic theory of fertility. Contingency table analyses show that legal migrants have an advantage over undocumented migrants in terms of background characteristics associated with higher paying work. On the whole, the legal migrants were older, slightly better educated and had been in the United States longer than the undocumented migrants. Legal status does increase both the male and female wage, but neither the male nor the female wage has a statistically significant effect on fertility, either directly or through the combination of both direct and indirect effects. Several of the sociological control variables entered into the equation did have statistically significant effects on fertility: mother's education; whether mother attended school in the U.S.; and mother's time of residence in the U.S.

18. Fan MYC. Socioeconomic status effects and ethnicity effects on fertility of Mexican Americans. Doctoral Dissertation, Los Angeles, California, University of California. 1980. 195 p. DAI; 41(1-A):414.

The author attempts to determine if fertility variation among members of an ethnic minority group can be attributed to socioeconomic characteristics or to cultural norms. Using data from a survey of **Mexican** Americans living in Los Angeles County, the author examines the effects on fertility of various factors, including woman's education, family income, husband's occupational status, wife's age, and age at marriage. The role of these influences as predictors of fertility is analyzed in relation to that of ethnic characteristics. Regression analysis, path analysis and multiple classification analysis all point out that even within an ethnic subculture of higher fertility, fertility and ethnic integration are negatively related when socioeconomic controls are introduced. Ethnicity does effect fertility apart from ethnicity's associations with socioeconomic and demographic factors. However, structural characteristics and demographic variables have a more important role, since factors like wife's age, age at marriage, education and nativity are better predictors of fertility than ethnicity characteristics.

19. Fischer NA ; Marcum JP. Ethnic integration, socioeconomic

status, and fertility among Mexican Americans. **Social Science Quarterly.** 1984;65(2):583-93.

The present research examines three hypotheses recently used to explain differential minority group fertility in the United States: the social characteristics hypothesis, the minority group status hypothesis, and a cultural factors hypothesis. The study sample is made up of **Mexican** American couples residing in Texas. In most instances, the results support the social characteristics hypothesis: that is, fertility is negatively associated with education such that neither the pattern of association nor the level is affected significantly by the degree of ethnic integration. Still, in at least one case, the results support the pronatalist norms part of the minority group status hypothesis. Fertility is negatively associated with education such that the level, but not the pattern of association, varies directly with the residential concentration of Mexican Americans. The finding that Mexican American couples residing in neighborhoods of Mexican American concentration have higher fertility than those residing elsewhere, supports arguments linking higher Mexican American fertility to pronatalist subcultural norms.

20. Ford K. Declining fertility rates of immigrants to the United States (with some exceptions). **Sociology and Social Research.** 1985;70(1):68-70.

This paper compiles 1970 and 1980 Census data on the fertility of immigrants to the United States from 20 countries or regions. The data show that: 1) immigrants are a heterogenous group with respect to fertility; 2) **Mexican** women have a higher fertility than other groups; and 3) most groups, including Mexican women, experienced the decline in fertility from 1970 to 1980 that was true of the native born population. Most immigrant groups have lower cumulative fertility and higher current fertility than native born women. This difference may mean that immigration delays childbearing. The very high fertility levels of some immigrant groups may be a cause for concern. Native born U.S. women, using the 1980 native born population as a standard, had 1.28 mean number of children ever born, Mexican women had 2.04 mean number of children, Central American women had 1.33, **Cuban** women had 1.01, and South American women had 1.12 mean number of children ever born.

21. Goldscheider C ; Uhlenberg PR. Minority group status and fertility. **American Journal of Sociology.** 1969;74:361-72.

Although this study did not include Hispanics, it is of significant theoretical importance for an understanding of the influence of minority group status on fertility. The authors postulate that the insecurities of minority group membership operate to depress fertility below majority levels when: 1) acculturation of minority group members has occurred in conjunction with the desire for acculturation; 2) equalization of social and economic characteristics occurs, particularly at middle and upper social class levels, and/or there is a desire for social and economic mobility; and 3) there is no pronatalist ideology associated with the minority group and no norm discouraging the use of efficient contraceptives. Analysis of minority group fertility suggests that previous explanations based on social and economic characteristics have been incomplete. The alternative hypothesis that, under given social and economic changes and concomitant acculturation, the insecurities and marginality associated with minority group status exert an independent effect on fertility appears consistent with the evidence.

22. Gurak DT. Assimilation and fertility: a comparison of Mexican American and Japanese American women. **Hispanic Journal of Behavioral Sciences.** 1980;2(3):219-39.

The sources of fertility differentials between two ethnic minority groups, one with low (Japanese), and one with high fertility (**Mexicans**), and majority whites are examined. Direct measures of assimilation have a net effect on fertility, with increases in assimilation being associated with a reduction in fertility for both minorities. The indicators of assimilation (residential segregation and intermarriage) operate similarly within each generation and for both ethnic groups. In fact, for Japanese American women, the social assimilation impact on fertility is greater among the native born women. Within the Japanese American population, which has low fertility levels, those women living in less ethnic neighborhoods have higher fertility than women in neighborhoods with high concentrations of foreign stock individuals. Similar results are obtained for the Mexican American population, which has high fertility. Those women living in neighborhoods with low concentrations of Hispanics have lower levels of fertility (consequently, more like the fertility levels of majority populations). While this analysis supports an assimilationist perspective, it also provides some support for the minority status thesis by documenting a nonlinear relationship between assimilation and fertility for Japanese Americans.

23. Gurak DT. Sources of ethnic fertility differences: an examination of five minority groups. **Social Science Quarterly.** 1978 Sep;59(2):295-310.

The author analyzes fertility data from the 1970 U.S. Census Public Use Sample for various ethnic groups. The population examined was 35 to 40 year old currently married women from six ethnic backgrounds: native white, native black, Japanese, **Cuban, Mexican,** and **Puerto Rican.** Analysis shows that fertility differentials between native whites and women from several low and high fertility groups cannot be explained by reference either to the social characteristics thesis or to the minority status thesis alone. Standardizing for differences in status and marital characteristics among groups does reduce fertility differentials, but only for Puerto Ricans does this reduction significantly narrow the gap with whites. Mexican fertility is high at all status levels, and there appears to exist an ethnically rooted tendency towards high fertility that does not appear, for the most part, to result from the common experience of belonging to a minority group. The extremely low fertility of Cuban women cannot be explained by references to differences with whites in social characteristics. The Cuban group differs from the others studied in an important respect: 97% are foreign born.

24. Halberstein RA. Fertility in two urban Mexican American populations. **Urban Anthropology.** 1976 Winter;5(4):335-50.

Mexican Americans are commonly described as exhibiting exceptionally high fertility levels and large completed families.

This generalization is explored in two urban Mexican American populations in the Kansas City metropolitan area. A demographic survey was administered to women of 88 households in Argentine and Armourdale Mexican American populations. Completed fertility in both populations, measured by the achieved reproduction (number of live births) of women aged 40 and older is lower than the Mexican American national average, and this is probably related to certain unique features of population structure and demographic dynamics. The two urbanized populations are geographically distinct from other Mexican Americans, and they are heterogeneous cosmopolitan communities rather than closed endogamous enclaves. This study supports the generally observed association between urbanization and fertility reduction. The author predicts that using the urban Mexican American populations of Argentine and Armourdale as models, completed Mexican American fertility in the future may not be strikingly different from the overall United States population.

25. Heath LL ; Roper BS ; King CD. A research note on children viewed as contributors to marital stability: the relationship to birth control use, ideal and expected family size. **Journal of Marriage and the Family.** 1974 May;36(2):304-6.

A tri-ethnic study of 120 working class blacks, Chicanos (**Mexicans**), and whites was employed to determine the contributions of children to marital satisfaction and stability together with differences in fertility. The data for this analysis were collected as part of a larger study of the relationship of various social/psychological factors to birth control use and family size. A multivariate analysis controlling for income indicated that ethnic or racial group membership and female employment were the primary sociocultural determinants of feelings toward children as high or low aids to family stability and satisfaction. It was found that belief in children as contributors to marital stability was significantly related to ideal family size and expected family size. The value was not directly related to contraceptive use, but did indicate a trend toward present use for those with low scores.

26. *Johnson CA. Mexican American women in the labor force and lowered fertility. **American Journal of Public Health.** 1976;66 (12):1186-8.

This study used 1970 Census data to examine the association between the participation of **Mexican** American women in the labor force and lowered fertility rates among these women. By using three dichotomized social characteristics: mother's education, labor force participation, and mother tongue, differing patterns of childbearing within this single ethnic group were identified. Results indicated that relationship of education to fertility was strongest among women under 20 years of age. The group which appears most likely to be able to achieve a controlled fertility pattern is composed of women in the labor force aged 20 to 34 years. The fact that the fertility of this group is more strongly associated with labor force participation than with education suggests that family planning programs should pay attention to the work careers of minority women, to locating family planning and other women's health services at the work place, and to utilization of work group associations as communication links.

27. Kazen PM ; Browning HL. Sociological aspects of the high

fertility of the United States Mexican-descent population: an
exploratory study. Austin, Texas, University of Texas, Population Research Center. 1967. 34 p.

The purpose of this article is to uncover those social factors
that help explain why fertility is so high among the **Mexican**-
descent United States population.   In 1964 a questionnaire was
administered to all Spanish surname households in a four block
area of Austin, Texas to obtain information on each family
member: name, age, place of birth, language spoken, years of
education, occupation, income, and religious affiliation.   The
main informant was the wife.   The investigation revealed that
the woman's full acceptance into society depends on her ability
to have and to care for many children. Despite this, most women
eventually desire to limit their family size.   Women rarely
discuss matters of sex or family planning, even with kin and
close friends.   Very few women, even those of higher socioeconomic status, have much knowledge about birth control techniques available to them, either prior to marriage or in early
marriage.   Along with sheer ignorance about these methods, false
perceptions exist about effectiveness and convenience of use.
Many are very reluctant even to attempt using mechanical devices.   When women really become concerned about limiting their
fertility they resort to sterilization.

28.   *Krubiner P.   Cultural factors in risk for adolescent pregnancy. Doctoral Dissertation, New York City, Yeshiva University.
October, 1982. 182 p. DAI;43(4-B):1258.

While a number of sociological and psychological correlates of
teenage pregnancy have been established, less is understood of
why these factors are related to a higher susceptibility to
unwanted pregnancy.   One objective of this study was to determine whether these personality and demographic characteristics
are similar for adolescents with the same pregnancy status, but
from different racial and cultural backgrounds. A second objective was to determine the effect of a previous abortion on the
adolescent's subsequent contraception decisions.   While black
and Hispanic adolescents from the inner city live in drastically
different environments than teenagers living in predominantly
white small town communities, adolescents from both environments
who became pregnant and carried to term had stikingly similar
characteristics.   Results of this study suggest that regardless
of ethnicity or environment, adolescents who carry to term come
from large families with low educational and occupational status, and often have experienced the death of a family member.

29.   Lee ES ; Roberts RE. Ethnic fertility differentials in the
southwest: the case of Mexican Americans reexamined. **Sociology
and Social Research**. 1981 Jan;65(2):194-210.

Fertility differentials among **Mexican** Americans and other ethnic
groups in the southwest are explored, based on the 1-in-1,000
Public Use Sample of the 1970 United States Census.   Particular
attention is given to refinement in defining the diverse population of Mexican Americans utilizing a combined objective/subjec-
tive criterion of Spanish surname and self-identification of
Spanish descent.   The two marginal groups identified by matching
these two identifiers exhibit an intermediate level of socioeconomic profiles and an intermediate level of fertility between
the Mexican American and Anglo groups, reflecting the gradual
process of acculturation, and an increasing trend toward inter-

marriage.   The results of more detailed analysis reveal that
socioeconomic factors exert different effects on fertility in
different ethnic groups and ethnic fertility differentials vary
at different stages of child progression, especially between
Mexican Americans and blacks,   suggesting different processes of
fertility transition between two minority groups.

30.   Linn MW ; Gurel L ; Carmichael J ; Weed P. Cultural comparisons of mothers with large and small families. **Journal of Bio-
social Science.** 1976;8:293-302.

Contraceptive knowledge and behavior of mothers of large (five
or more children) and small (under three children) families in
four subcultures were compared with white Protestants.   Four
hundred and forty-nine mothers aged 30 to 45 years were studied
from black, **Cuban,** Indian, **Mexican,** and white groups.   With
social class, knowledge of birth control, and degree of religiosity held constant,   the best predictors of family size were
the mother's desired family size (expressed as desired minus
actual children), age at childbirth, and age at marriage. Data
suggest that family size is not purely a function of birth
control knowledge, but related to early marriage and pregnancy,
and in keeping with attitudes about an ideal family size.   In
general, factors related to size were stronger in the white
group than in the other groups. In a few instances certain
cultures were not consistent with others in overall trends. Any
intervention program needs to be aware of differences in motivation that arise from cultural influence.

31.   Lopez DE ; Sabagh G. Untangling structural and normative
aspects of the minority status fertility hypothesis. **American
Journal of Sociology.** 1978;83(6):1 & 491-7.

A persistent problem in the analysis of fertility variation in
the United States has been the nature and extent of ethnic and
minority fertility differentials and the degree to which they
can be accounted for by socioeconomic factors.   Residual minority fertility left after the usual socioeconomic correlates of
fertility are controlled is usually attributed to cultural differences.   But such residuals can be attributed just as well to
structural factors.   Since the residual differential fertility
of racial and ethnic minorities can be explained in theoretically opposed ways, effects due to subcultural norms can be
established only by direct measurement.   Data from a recent
survey of 1,129 Los Angeles **Mexican** couples indicate that ethnic
integration is actually associated with reduced fertility, suggesting that the structural negative minority status effect on
fertility hypothesized by Goldscheider and Uhlenberg operates
even within a high fertility minority group.   This contradicts
their suggestion that high minority fertility is due to subcultural norms.

32.   Marcum JP ; Bean FD. Ethnic status as a factor in the relationship between mobility and fertility: the Mexican American
case. **Social Forces.** 1976 Sep;55(1):135-48.

This paper sets forth contrasting hypotheses about the influence
of racial and ethnic group membership on the relationship between mobility and fertility.   One may be termed the minority
group status approach, and the other the underdevelopment approach.   Both perspectives offer bases for predicting fertility
levels that deviate from the average levels typical of persons

from particular social strata. However, the former implies greater fertility deviations the more integrated the minority group is into the larger society, whereas the latter suggests greater deviations the less integrated the minority group is into the larger society. These ideas are tested using data from a sample of **Mexican** American couples, split according to generational distance from Mexico. The results indicate more support for the minority group status than the underdevelopment hypothesis. This was revealed by lower than average expected fertility on the part of couples removed at least three generations from Mexico.

33. *Michael RT ; Tuma NB. Entry into marriage and parenthood by young men and women: the influence of family background. **Demography.** 1985 Nov;22(4):515-44.

The authors investigate the influence of family background on early entry into marriage and parenthood among white, Hispanic, and black men and women aged 14 to 22 in the first (1979) wave of the National Longitudinal Survey of Youth. Family background is highly associated with early entry into marriage for whites of both genders and female Hispanics, and also with early entry into parenthood for all groups except black males. Large group differences in family characteristics explain most of the differences between white and Hispanic women in early marriage and parenthood, and about half the differences in early parenthood between black and white women, but do not explain the observed variations among other race/gender groups.

34. Mookherjee HN. Differential fertility and minority status. Paper presented at the Annual Meeting of the Rural Sociological Society, College Station, Texas. August 22-25, 1984. 19 p.

This paper tests the minority status hypothesis for interpreting interethnic and interracial fertility differences in the United States. To determine the intergroup variation in number of children born to a family, black Americans, Hispanic Americans and American Indians are compared to American whites. The influence of minority status on the number of children born is examined by determining the compositional differences between the minority and white populations. Data are taken from the 1970 Public Use Samples for the U.S., the unit of analysis being married couples. The results suggest that minority status has an independent effect on fertility. The pattern of differences in regression coefficients was generally consistent with the idea that minority status is an important consideration in determining fertility. These findings suggest that minority group status certainly produces tensions which may also increase fertility, instead of reducing it. The authors argue that the subcultural norms of the minority groups under study (blacks, Hispanics, and Indians) are distinct and the group members may not desire to be assimilated totally, but desire socioeconomic mobility.

35. *Mott FL. Early fertility behavior among American youth: evidence from the 1982 National Longitudinal Survey of Labor Force Behavior of Youth. Presented at the 1983 Annual Meeting of the American Public Health Association, Dallas, Texas. November, 1983.

This paper examines the sexuality and fertility behavior of American adolescents based on data from the 1982 National Longi-

tudinal Survey of Labor Force Behavior of Youth.   The author
identifies which background characteristics and attitudes appear
to predict sexual activity, contraceptive use, fertility behavior and the desire for early fertility.   For young never married
women, factors including church attendance, living with two
parents, having a traditional orientation regarding female sex
roles, expecting postgraduate education, and higher measured
intelligence were significant predictors of less sexual activity.   Also, drug and alcohol use showed a strong positive
association with sexual activity.   With the exception of the
nontraditionality measure, all of these factors were also significant predictors for younger men.   Furthermore, there is marginal evidence that young women with greater self esteem are
less sexually active, (but contracept better if they are sexually active), less likely to have an early birth, but more likely
to have wanted the pregnancy if they had it.   From the racial
and ethnic perspective, even after controlling for the various
socioeconomic factors in the model, black male and female respondents had above average levels of sexual activity. Young
Hispanic males were also above average in this regard, while
Hispanic females were significantly below average.   The pattern-
ing of the overall results suggests strongly the importance of
socialization and social/psychological considerations as fertility behavior determinants.

36.   *Mott FL. The pace of early childbearing among young American mothers. Paper prepared under a contract with the Employment
and Training Administration, U.S. Department of Labor. (Unpublished) 1985. 18 p.

This paper presents basic data on early repeat childbearing for
young women maturing in the late 1970s and early 1980s and
suggests which factors are most closely associated with repeat-
ing the early birth.   This study uses data from the National
Longitudinal Survey of Work Experience of Youth, a nationally
representative longitudinal sample of 6,288 females and 6,398
males aged 14 to 22 when first interviewed in 1979.   The sample
was interviewed on an annual basis through 1984.   Results are
presented in tables and charts and discussed throughout the
article.   Taking all races together including **Mexicans, Puerto
Ricans** and **Cubans,** almost one-third of the women who had a first
birth before their sixteenth birthday had a second birth within
24 months.   Increasing age at first birth is predictive of a
greater delay in subsequent childbearing.   For all ages at first
birth, the Hispanic mother appears more likely to bear a second
child more rapidly than either her black or white counterpart.
The following factors were significantly associated with childbearing before age 17:   church attendance, maternal education,
and coming from a stable (two parent) background.   These were
associated with below average probabilities of having an early
first birth.

37.   *Powers MG ; Gurak DT ; Macisco JJ Jr ; Tanfer K ; Weller
RH. Influence of life experiences at or prior to marriage on the
early fertility of Puerto Rican and Dominican women.   Presented
at the 56th Annual Meeting of the Population Association of
America, San Francisco, California. April 3-5, 1986.

This study focuses on the influence of factors at or prior to
first marriage on selected measures of the fertility of **Puerto
Rican** and **Dominican** women.   The data contain detailed retrospective life histories, and a life-course model is used to test

hypotheses about the causal processes which determine fertility. This preliminary analysis examines the effects of factors exist- ing in the women's life experiences at or prior to the first marital union, on the total number of children born in the five years after entry into the union, and the probability of having a child during the first two years of a union. As might be expected, based on previous research, the most important predic- tors of having a birth within the first two years of a legal union are education related variables. There are no period effects on the timing of the first birth. Several variables affect the number of births within five years of the start of a legal union: employment in the 18 months prior to first union, number of births prior to marriage, education, and period of first union. When all first unions are examined, the results differ from those for first legal unions. The results for Puerto Rican and Dominican women are compared to findings from similar analyses of a 1974 follow-up of 1957 and 1958 graduates of Illinois high schools, a sample of predominantly white, non-Hispanic women.

38. *Robbins C ; Kaplan HB ; Martin SS. Antecedents of preg- nancy among unmarried adolescents. **Journal of Marriage and the Family.** 1985;47(3):567-83.

Using data from a 1971 survey of seventh grade students in Texas, multivariate causal models were tested to predict out-of- wedlock adolescent pregnancy. Among the males, having a girl- friend become pregnant is associated with school difficulties, low parental socioeconomic status, and high popularity. Among females, pregnancy risk is related to race (black women more likely than white women to experience early nonmarital preg- nancy; Hispanic women are less likely), low socioeconomic sta- tus, father absence, number of siblings, school difficulties, family stress, and popularity. The 1981-83 follow-up study found 26% of the women, but only 15% of the men reporting that they (or their girlfriends) had experienced adolescent pregnan- cies. The analyses do not support culture-of-poverty assump- tions. Powerlessness is weakly related to the 18 to 20 year old males' involvement in nonmarital pregnancies. Surprisingly, it was found that powerlessness is inversely related to pregnancy risk for girls in father present families, possibly because girls who feel powerless may be more submissive to parental authority that discourages sexual activity.

39. *Roberts RE ; Lee ES. Minority group status and fertility revisited. **American Journal of Sociology.** 1974 Sep;o0(2):503-23.

This paper examines the relationship between minority group status and fertility in five southwestern states (Ari- zona, California, Colorado, New Mexico, and Texas) with the basic data source coming from the 1-in-100 Public Use Sample of the 1960 Census. The data are confined to women who were married before the age of 25 and were not employed at the time of the census. Findings reveal that the fertility rate is higher for rural than for urban residents, lower socio- economic groups, non-whites, minority categories, and higher for the blacks and those with a Spanish surname. The cumula- tive fertility of Spanish surnamed women aged 40 to 49 in 1960 was consistently higher than that of black and other white women at every level of comparison. The differential tends to be wider at the lower socioeconomic level in rural areas than at the higher socioeconomic level in urban areas.

The fertility differential by occupation among Spanish surnamed women is not as pronounced as that by education in both urban and rural areas. It was also shown that certain structural variables such as income, place of residence, occupation, education, etc. did not provide an explanation for fertility differentials.

40. Sabagh G ; Lopez D. Religiosity and fertility: the case of Chicanas. **Social Forces.** 1980 Dec;59(2):431-9.

Data from a probability sample of 1,129 Chicanas (**Mexican** American women) married to Chicanos and interviewed in Los Angeles in 1973 were used to analyze the effects of religious norms on the fertility of Catholic women 35 to 44 years old in the sample. The assessment of the effects of religious norms are based on measures of religiosity and religious participation. The findings indicate that if religiosity is a measure of adherence to the norms of the Roman Catholic Church, then these norms have a net impact on the fertility of Chicanas reared in the United States, but not on the fertility of those brought up in Mexico. The other independent variables in the multiple regression analysis include indices of socioeconomic status, a scale of sociocultural ethnicity, two measures of ghettoization, and age at marriage. The findings imply that the characteristics of the country of upbringing have to be taken into account in any analyses of the effects of religious norms on the reproductive behavior of Catholics.

41. Schoen R. Toward a theory of the demographic implications of ethnic stratification. **Social Science Quarterly.** 1978 Dec;59 (3):468-81.

In ethnically stratified societies, some lower socioeconomic groups are able to move into a middle class status while others are not. In this essay the author refutes Uhlenberg's (1972) comparison of **Mexican** Americans and Japanese Americans, where he concluded that differences in the economic success of those groups could be related to differences in their demographic behavior. One can argue, however, that Japanese Americans, but not Mexican Americans could move into a middle niche, and that the demographic patterns of the two groups are best seen as consequences rather than causes of their social and economic circumstances. For Mexican Americans to have achieved the same degree of rapid social mobility as Japanese Americans would thus have involved profound social and economic changes for the larger society, and it is difficult to see how such changes could have been brought about by a change in the demographic behavior of Mexican Americans. These considerations do not mean that demographic behavior does not influence social and economic mobility, but they do challenge Uhlenberg's contention that the two groups started on a roughly equal footing, and that the larger society was less favorable for Japanese Americans than for Mexican Americans.

42. *Slesinger DP ; Okada Y. Fertility patterns of Hispanic migrant farm women: testing the effect of assimilation. **Rural Sociology.** 1984;49(3):430-40.

A ten percent stratified random sample survey of Hispanic migrant farm women in Wisconsin indicates that these women have greater numbers of children than other United States women. The degree of assimilation into the mainstream culture, measured by

whether or not the women spoke English, was inversely related to
fertility.   Statistical   regression analysis revealed that   age
was   the   variable most strongly associated with   birth   number,
followed by educational status.   Forty-five percent of the older
women   were   illiterate,   compared with 15% of the younger women.
Only   three   percent of the older women and 12% of   the   younger
women had completed high school.   Migrant women who spoke   only
Spanish had borne, on average, one more child than had women who
were   bilingual.   Child mortality experience was   considerable:
15%   of   the women had experienced a death of one or   more   live
births.   Over a third of the women had never used any contraceptive method.   Of the 42% now using contraception, 29% had an IUD
in place,   while over half used oral contraceptives.   Fewer than
20%   of   the women said they would like more   information   about
family planning.

43.   *Sorenson AM.   Fertility expectations and ethnic   identity
among   Mexican American adolescents: an expression of   cultural
ideals. **Sociological Perspectives.** 1985 Jul;28(3):339-50.

Survey data from Arizona secondary schools were used to test the
applicability   of structural and minority status   hypotheses   to
the   differential fertility expectations of **Mexican** American and
Anglo adolescents. The fertility expectations of these Anglo and
Mexican   American   respondents   parallel   the   expectations   of
adults.   Analyses   of the number of children expected by   these
respondents,   and   their implied parity progression ratios,   indicate   that   indices   of acculturation are   more   important   in
explaining   expected   fertility than are   measures   of   parental
socioeconomic   status   or respondent's expected   status.   Among
Mexican American respondents language spoken at   home,   nativity
of   the   respondent   and his or her father,   and   residence   are
associated with expected fertility.   These indices of acculturation retain their importance even when father's   education,   father's occupation, and number of siblings are introduced.

44.   *Sorenson AM.   Structural and cultural effects on the fertility   expectations of Mexican American and Anglo   adolescents.
Paper   of the American Sociological   Association.   (Unpublished)
1984.

Survey   data gathered in Arizona secondary schools were used   to
test   the applicability of structural and cultural hypotheses to
the differential fertility expectations of 1,955 **Mexican** American and Anglo adolescents.   The structural hypothesis was tested
using   the   respondents'   educational and occupational   expectations,   and father's educational attainment.   The results indicate   that   these   structural variables do not account   for   the
higher   fertility expectations of Mexican American   respondents.
The   cultural hypothesis was also tested among Mexican   American
respondents.   Variables   representing ethnic identity   such   as
speaking   Spanish   at   home and the birth of the   respondent   or
his/her   father in Mexico are associated with   higher   fertility
expectations   in this group.   These cultural variables retained
their significance even when father's occupation was   introduced
as   an additional measure of socioeconomic effects and with   the
addition   of   number of siblings using minimum logit   chi-square
regression.   Other cultural variables examined have no significant effect on fertility expectations.

45.   Swicegood CG. **Language, opportunity costs and Mexican American fertility.** Austin, Texas, University of Texas. 1982. 198 p.

The research utilizes data from the 1976 Survey of Income and Education which was based on a stratified, multistage cluster sample of approximately 151,200 households in the United States. The research purpose was to test certain hypotheses concerning patterns of childbearing within the **Mexican** American population. It was found that English proficiency and frequent use of English were negatively associated with the cumulative fertility of Mexican American women in 1976 and that these relationships held after controlling for a number of sociodemographic variables. These language factors interacted with female education in their effect on fertility. For the total sample of Mexican American women, and for the foreign born subsample, bilingualism had no statistically significant net association with fertility, but for native born women bilingualism was related to higher levels of childbearing when included in the same model with proficiency. Most puzzling was the net positive relationship between English proficiency and fertility when the variable for bilingualism was included in the regression model for native born women.

46. Swicegood CG ; Stephen EH ; Opitz W ; Cardenas G. Language usage and fertility in the Mexican origin population: results from the 1980 Census. Presented at the 56th Annual Meeting of the Population Association of America, San Francisco, California. April 3-5, 1986.

This paper uses 1980 Census data to examine the relationship between English language usage and fertility among the ever married **Mexican** origin women in the United States. Within every five year age grouping of women aged 20 to 44, the mean number of children ever born decreases with greater English language proficiency. The authors also found that the negative impact of education on fertility is much more pronounced for women with the greatest English proficiency. Both of these patterns vary in interpretable ways according to the age and nativity of the respondent. The results are discussed in terms of the opportunity structures encountered by Mexican origin and other minority group women.

47. Szapocznik J ; Scopetta MA ; Kurtines W. Theory and measurement of acculturation. **Inter-American Journal of Psychology.** 1978;12:113-30.

This paper outlines a psychosocial model of acculturation intended to account for the occurrence of intergenerational/acculturational differences in immigrant families including **Cubans.** Two acculturation scales were developed measuring self-reported behaviors and value dimensions. The behavioral scale provided a highly reliable and valid measure of acculturation and proved superior to the value scale in almost every respect. Behavioral and value acculturation were found to be linear functions of the amount of time a person was exposed to the host culture. The rate at which the behavioral acculturation process took place was found to be a function of the age and sex of the individual. The findings suggest that intergenerational/acculturational differences develop because younger members of the family acculturate more rapidly than older family members.

48. Tienda M. The Mexican American population. In: Hawley AH and Mazie SM, eds. **Nonmetropolitan America in transition.** Chapel Hill, North Carolina, University of North Carolina Press. 1981.

p. 502-48. (Institute for Research in Social Science, Monograph Series).

This paper summarizes data from various sources concerning socioeconomic and demographic circumstances of Chicanos residing in rural and nonmetropolitan areas. In regard to fertility, the author points out that historically and currently Chicano women have higher fertility than any other Spanish origin group as well as the black population. A number of factors have contributed to the persistence of high fertility among **Mexican** American women. Among the most commonly noted are differences in socioeconomic status, younger marriage, closer birth spacing intervals, minority status, and offspring gender, but these factors are insufficient to account completely for observed differentials. An additional factor thought to have produced high fertility is family size norms. Several consequences of sustained high fertility are a relatively young population with a large share of individuals in dependent ages and large families.

49. *Uhlenberg P. Fertility patterns within the Mexican American population. **Social Biology.** 1973 Mar;20(1):30-9.

When standardized for rural/urban residence, **Mexican** Americans have a higher fertility rate than any other racial or ethnic group in the United States. Among women in urban areas between the ages of 35 and 49, the average number of children for Mexican Americans is 50% greater than for blacks and about 70% greater than for native whites. Yet, within the Mexican American population, the middle class has the same size families as other whites. Without information on desired family size, it cannot be determined to what extent the high fertility of the lower class results from their desire for large families or from their inability to prevent unwanted pregnancies. Future trends in Mexican American fertility are most likely to be associated with how rapidly the group accomplishes upward social mobility and increased involvement in U.S. society, although family planning services will possibly have some effect. Mexican Americans have become more and more dissatisfied with their disadvantaged circumstances, and their efforts to change existing conditions may directly affect their reproductive behavior.

50. Warren CW. Determinants of Mexican American fertility. Presented at the 52nd Annual Meeting of the Population Association of America, Pittsburgh, Pennsylvania. April 14-16, 1983. (Unpublished) 35 p.

The focus of this study was on which intermediate variables are most important as determinants of **Mexican** American fertility, and do these variables help clarify the previously found negative relationship between years of schooling and fertility. Bongaarts' model of the four intermediate variables which directly effect fertility is presented. Results showed a pattern similar to that expected by Bongaarts (1983) who stated that a typical transition from natural to controlled fertility is accompanied by a shortening of postpartum infecundability, a large increase in contraceptive use, and a decline in the proportion married. For the groups closest to natural fertility (Mexico National and Mexico Six Northern States), lactation, contraception, and marriage all were moderately important as intermediate variables. For the groups closest to controlled fertility (United States whites and Anglos) contraceptive use was a very

important fertility inhibiting factor.   Marriage was important,
but not nearly as important as contraception, and induced abortion was moderately important.   For the two Mexican American
groups contraceptive use was an important intermediate variable
and marriage was a moderately important factor.

2. Sex-Related Attitudes
and Knowledge

Some controversy surrounds the study of attitudes of Hispanics in the United States. In particular, a number of authors
have criticized popular and research stereotypes of Hispanic
families as authoritarian, male-dominated, and more traditional
on the whole range of sex-related attitudes. Such sweeping
generalizations are clearly unfounded. In fact, on many measures Hispanics appear to hold attitudes which are similar to
those of other U.S. adults with similar background characteristics.

Studies of ethnic differences in attitudes are particularly
hindered by the lack of uniformity of definitions, (particularly
of such terms as "machismo" or "familism"), and by the need for
studies which control for such important background variables as
socioeconomic status, education and country of origin.

In addition to **authoritarianism, machismo, and general
family values,** other variables measured in studies abstracted
here include **husband/wife communication** and attitudes toward **sex
roles, decision-making, value of children, family size, pregnancy, abortion, contraception, and rape.** Of these, perhaps the
most consistent findings have been the higher family size
desires of Hispanic adults.

Far fewer studies have been done of sex-related knowledge
among Hispanics. In studies of adolescents researchers have
applied measures of **knowledge of sex, knowledge of natality,** and
reports of parent/child conversations about sex.

51. *Abramson PR ; Moriuchi KD ; Waite MS ; Perry LB. Parental
attitudes about sexual education: cross-cultural differences and
covariate controls. **Archives of Sexual Behavior.** 1983 Oct;12(5):
381-97.

This study examines cross-cultural differences in parental attitudes and experiences regarding childhood sexual education.
Parents with children ranging in age from one to ten were in-

cluded in the study from four cultural groups: of the 87 couples, all Americans, 22 were **Mexican**, 20 Black, 27 Caucasian,
and 18 Japanese in background.   Mexican American parents expressed the most discomfort discussing such issues as masturba-
tion, intercourse and nudity with their children, suggesting a
pattern of cultural effects. However, an analysis of covariance
indicated that husband's education was related to each of these
findings rather than cultural differences.   In general, the
most salient and consistent finding of the investigation is the
pronounced significance of the covariate controls.   Although a
few cross-cultural effects remained significant despite the
influence of a covariate, most of the findings were biased by a
concomitant demographic variable, such as father's education or
mother's religiosity.

52. Alcalay R. Hispanic women in the United States: family and
work relations. **Migration Today**. 1984;12(3):13-20.

This study reviews research and data on the factors influencing
the lives of Hispanic women in the United States.   Differences
are considered between **Mexican** American, **Puerto Rican**, and **Cuban**
American women, and between Anglo and Hispanic family norms.
While considerable differences exist between Hispanic groups in
the U.S. there are important common elements.   One of the most
significant is the extended family.   Within the extended family
setting, the Hispanic woman derives a great deal of culturally
sanctioned power and authority from her role as wife and mother.
A significant difference in Anglo and Latin norms about motherhood and child care is reflected in social legislation.   Although Latin women face considerable social difficulties in
entering the work force, nevertheless, economic necessity has
forced a significant percentage of Latin women to obtain employment.

53. Alcalay R ; Caldiz L. Barrier to effective intercultural
communication in family planning. Paper presented at the Speech
Communications Association Intercultural Communication Conference, Honolulu, Hawaii. August 4, 1979. (Washington, D.C., Educational Resources Information Center).

The focus of this article is the communication problems between
Anglo American family planning counselors and their Latin American clients in a rural community in California.   Cultural differences in attitudes toward family, work, and sexuality were
examined.   For the Latin American woman the extended family
provides her with a positive self-identity and serves as a
source of social relations.   In addition, it favors and facilitates raising a large number of children.   The family structure
in the United States, in contrast, is nuclear; the woman is
socially isolated if she remains solely in the role of housewife.   Also, because of the absence of the extended family, the
child rearing task is the responsibility of the couple. For the
Anglo American woman, work becomes a source of identity, influence and social relations.   In almost all Latin American countries labor laws make it easier for women to have and bring up
children than the legislation in North America.   The risk of
unwanted pregnancies is greater for Latin American women because
of cultural obstacles, such as the Catholic Church, to information on sexual matters.

54. Alvirez D. The effects of formal church affiliation and
religiosity on the fertility patterns of Mexican American Catho-

lics. **Demography**. 1973 Feb;10(1):19-36.

The effects of religion on the fertility patterns of **Mexican** Americans are examined with two different path models, the Institutional Model using formal affiliation with the Roman Catholic Church as a measure of religion, and the Religiosity Model using a measure of religiosity. Each model, tested separately for husbands and wives, examines the effects of religion on types of contraceptive methods used and on wanted family size. Although the majority of Mexican Americans are Catholics and tend to have large families, religion does not seem to have the same effect on their fertility patterns as on that of other Catholics in the United States. Among the men, neither formal affiliation nor religiosity affect the fertility patterns in any way, while among the women, the effect is slight. Considering the Catholic church's position on contraceptive usage, it is especially noteworthy that religion does not affect the use or non-use of the more effective means of contraception, a factor contributing to the generally weak association between the measures of religion and wanted family size. The last section attempts a partial explanation of why the results turned out as they did.

55. Amaro HD. Psychosocial determinants of abortion attitudes among Mexican American women. Doctoral Dissertation, Los Angeles, California, University of California. 1981. 247 p. DAI;43(10-B):3404.

Data were gathered through structured interviews with 137 **Mexican** American women seeking general health care in a community health care clinic. The overwhelming majority of Mexican American women approved of abortion for medical reasons, one-third approved of abortion for social reasons. Demographic (education, occupation, age) and psychosocial (religiosity, acculturation, marital status, sexual activity, attitudes toward sex roles, childbearing, contraceptives, prior experience with abortion) variables were found to be associated with abortion attitudes. Components of the Fishbein-Ajzen model contributed differently to the prediction of abortion intentions depending on whether the reason for abortion was medical or social. Contrary to the model stipulations, variables other than the model components had a direct influence on the behavioral intention to have an abortion for medical reasons. While Mexican American women's abortion attitudes are similar to those of other Americans reported in previous studies, there are culturally specific characteristics which shape their attitudes. Further, the antecedents of abortion attitudes and probably of the abortion decision-making process itself are markedly different under medical and social circumstances.

56. Andrade SJ. Family roles of Hispanic women: stereotypes, empirical findings and implications for research. Revised version of a paper presented at the Hispanic Women's Conference, Hispanic Research Center, New York City, Fordham University. (Unpublished) November, 1980. 22 p.

Three major research initiatives are highlighted: 1) the need to acknowledge the enormous heterogeneity of Hispanics (**Mexican** Americans, **Puerto Ricans**) in the United States and the different political historical circumstances affecting different groups. Research should be developed within a sophisticated elaboration of internal colonialism theory to reflect more accurately the conditions of these groups, particularly with respect to family roles and relations; 2) social science field methodology to include a greater emphasis on observation, measurement and analysis of actual family behaviors or of indicators closer to those behaviors than the retrospective self-reports and written questionnaires which focus too heavily on values and attitudes; and 3) the need for interdisciplinary, multi-method programs of research to assess behavioral interactions between institutions or organizations and Hispanics as consumers and staff members. There has been too great a reliance on attempts to measure characteristics of Hispanics in isolation from their ecological settings.

57. Andrade SJ. Social science stereotypes of the Mexican American woman: policy implications for research. **Hispanic Journal of Behavioral Sciences**. 1982;4(2):223-44.

Reviewing the social science literature on the Chicana or **Mexican** American woman reveals a tenaciously perpetuated stereotype in which she appears almost exclusively as a submissive maternal figure. The size and selection of many of the samples are questionable for purposes of generalizing to the entire population. The main concern is to what extent social scientists and the media are dictating norms to the Chicano family and to what extent are social planners and educators being influenced by these images. Examples from three distinct areas of research conclude with interpretations of Mexican American women that differ considerably from those with a heavy emphasis on cultural values: 1) demographic analyses of the 1970 Public Use Samples of the Census that acknowledge the disadvantaged economic position of Mexican Americans; 2) studies that are beginning to measure empirically the family dynamics of Mexican Americans; and 3) family planning studies that attempt to examine the interaction between health care delivery systems and Mexican American contraceptive behavior.

58. *Andrade SJ ; Torres MG. Aspirations of adolescent Hispanic females for marriage, children, education, and employment. Final report to the Hispanic Youth Employment Research Center, Washington, D.C., National Council of La Raza. May, 1982. 191 p.

This final report includes two documents: "Young Hispanics in the United States, their aspirations for the future," and "Young Hispanic mothers enrolled in school and/or employed, interviewed in the 1979 National Longitudinal Survey." The goal of the first paper is to provide descriptive profiles of the marriage, childbearing, educational and occupational aspirations of adolescent Hispanic females and males, and an analysis of the relative differences and similarities between young **Mexicans, Puerto Ricans** and **Cubans,** and the other major racial and ethnic groups in our society. The findings focus primarily on the interaction between sex and ethnicity in terms of its effect on young people's perception of their ability to achieve. The second paper documents the findings of the Hispanic, black, and white working and/or studying mothers' NLS subsample analysis. A profile of the young Hispanic working/enrolled mother is presented, focusing on education, occupation, childbearing and family role attitudes.

59. *Bassoff BZ ; Ortiz ET. Teen women: disparity between cognitive values and anticipated life events. **Child Welfare.** 1984 Mar/Apr;63(2):125-38.

Aspirations for a good education, financial independence, a good marriage or relationship, and self-worth emerged as the most important values for the teen women questioned in this study conducted in 1981 as part of a multi-year research and demonstration project. The program is sponsored by private foundations and is administered by the Center for Women's Studies and Services, San Diego, California. Five hundred and fifty-seven young women enrolled in three high schools with high dropout and early pregnancy rates were interviewed. For young black women, good education, financial independence, and self-worth were more highly valued. Hispanics and Asians varied from the total group in that they gave a lower value to all dimensions tested, with the exception of education. It is the position of the authors of this paper that learned helplessness is a pertinent factor which can be used to explain the failure of some young women to prevent early pregnancy. A variety of programs and services can provide the vehicle for learning mastery over one's life. Overall goals should be to expand choices and provide alternatives to young women regarding the direction of their life.

60. Bean FD ; Curtis RL Jr ; Marcum JP. Familism and marital satisfaction among Mexican Americans: the effects of family size, wife's labor force participation, and conjugal power. **Journal of Marriage and the Family.** 1977 Nov;39(4):759-67.

The concept of familism as an important aspect of **Mexican** American family life is studied by examining the effects of three variables on marital satisfaction: family size, wife's participation in the labor force, and conjugal power. A reanalysis was conducted on data gathered from 325 Mexican American couples in 1969 through the Austin Family Survey. Results revealed that: 1) husbands and wives are more satisfied with the affective side of their marriage when there are fewer children and when the conjugal power structure is more egalitarian; 2) husbands are less satisfied when the wife works; and 3) wives are less satisfied when they work voluntarily. When the sample is split according to occupation, the pattern of labor force participation effects is found to hold only among lower class couples, suggesting that class rather than ethnicity is the more important factor conditioning the relationship. Findings indicate the levels of marital satisfaction are a product of marital conditions per se more than of culturally based values about familism.

61. *Becerra R ; Fielder E. Adolescent attitudes and behavior. **Institute for Social Science Research Quarterly.** 1985 Nov;1(2): 4-7.

This paper reports on a survey of 1,000 adolescent females from Los Angeles County. The discussion outlines preliminary descriptive findings on the differences in sexual attitudes and behavior among sexually active and not sexually active **Mexican** American and white adolescents, aged 13 to 19. Sociodemographically, the families of the Mexican and Anglo teenagers were distinctly different. The Mexican American adolescents were less likely than the whites to be in school and more likely to come from low socioeconomic status homes. In general, sexually active Mexican daughters came from more acculturated families. The nonsexually active Mexican daughters are more likely to come from a home where the primary spoken language is Spanish. The sexually active Mexican Americans are more likely than whites to perceive themselves in a committed relationship, and more likely

to have had only one sexual partner.   For this reason, many may
not feel the necessity to use contraception, both for religious
reasons   and   because   they have plans to marry   the   young   man
anyway.   Children   are viewed as central to a family commitment
and are a welcomed addition.   While premarital sex is not   con-
doned,   and there is still a high premium placed on virginity in
Hispanic communities, the process of acculturation and a variety
of other life circumstances has modified these cultural mores.

62.   Bird   HR   ;   Canino G.   The Puerto Rican   family: cultural
factors and family intervention strategies. **Journal of the American Academy of Psychoanalysis.** 1982 Apr;10(2):257-68.

The   composition of the family,   the important role of   the   extended family, the impact of machismo, the authoritarian pattern
of   child   rearing,   and the religious practices of   the   **Puerto
Rican**   family have been documented through the findings reported
by   other researchers.   It is noted that the high rate of   back
and   forth migration between Puerto Rico and   the   mainland,   as
well as the colonial status of the society,   creates a situation
of   accelerated   change and shifting cultural patterns.   It   is
important   to   point out the normative patterns on   the   island.
Quite often a well intentioned clinician,   when confronted   with
issues   such   as   exaggerated machismo or certain   responses   to
stress,   may   tend   to dismiss them as purely cultural   and   not
address   the real issues leading to dysfunction or   utilize   the
most appropriate treatment modality.   Structural family therapy
as   a   particularly   useful treatment modality is   discussed   at
length,   and   its   applicability and the justification for   its
utilization in families under stress is   elaborated.   Treatment
strategies   and their relationship to Puerto Rican family structure is delineated.

63.   *Borup   JH.   Sex standards of college students: double   or
single?   **International Journal of Sociology of the Family.**   1973
Sep;3(2):217-24.

This   study used a sample of 480 college freshmen to assess   sex
standards   regarding   acceptable levels of intimacy   at   various
stages   of   courtship.   No significant differences   were   found
between   the standards of Catholic Anglo Americans and   Catholic
Mexican Americans or between Catholics and   Protestants.   There
were significant differences, however, between the sexes, in the
expected   direction.   The   author   concludes that there   is   no
longer a strong double standard of sexual behavior.

64.   *Borus ME   ;   Crowley JE   ;   Rumberger RW   ;   Santos R   ;   Shapiro
D.   Pathways to the future: a longitudinal study of young Ameri-
cans.   Preliminary   report,   youth and the labor   market,   1979.
Columbus,   Ohio,   Ohio State University,   Center for Human Resource
Research. (Unpublished) 1980.

This monograph presents preliminary cross-tabulation analyses of
the   1979   National Longitudinal Survey of   Youth   Labor   Market
Experiences   of 12,693 youth,   aged 14 to 21.   Hispanic,   non-
Hispanic,   black,   and   non-Hispanic non-black,   poor youth were
oversampled.   Chapters address: 1) demographic and socioeconomic   characteristics of the youth in this age cohort;   2)   youth
employment   status;   3) youth employment conditions   (jobs);   4)
youth   employment patterns (1978);   5) government sponsored   employment and training programs;   6) working students;   7)   youth
not   in   school   or the labor force;   8) job turnovers   and   job

leavers; 9) job search activities; 10) perceptions of discrimination and barriers to employment; 11) willingness to work; 12) health status of youth; 13) attitudes toward school; 14) educational aspirations and expectations; 15) experience of high school students according to variations in their curriculum; 16) high school dropouts; 17) college students population; 18) first job after leaving school; 19) desire for occupational training; 20) aspirations for age 35; 21) ideal, desired, and expected fertility; 22) attitudes toward women working, fertility expectations, and their relation to educational and occupational expectations; 23) knowledge of world of work; and 24) influences on life decisions.

65. Cochrane SH ; Bean FD. Husband/wife differences in the demand for children. **Journal of Marriage and the Family.** 1976 May;38(2):297-307.

The presence or absence of differences between husbands and wives in patterns of relationship between certain economic variables and desired family size may indicate: 1) whether or not conjugal roles condition the effects of economic factors on the demand for children; and 2) the extent to which assumptions in economic models of fertility about the nature and existence of common family utility functions are empirically supported.   In order to test for such differences, equations regressing husband's and wife's desired family size separately on selected economic, social, and background variables are estimated using data from a survey of **Mexican** American couples.   The results reveal considerable husband/wife differences in patterns of relationship, particularly in the cases of variables measuring wife's wage and labor force participation.   Further analysis reveals that whether husband's desired family size is affected primarily by the wife's potential wage or by her current labor force participation depends on the degree to which the wife has mutually acknowledged influence on family decisions concerning the number of children to have.

66. Cooney RS ; Rogler LH ; Hurrel RM ; Ortiz V. Decision-making in intergenerational Puerto Rican families. **Journal of Marriage and the Family.** 1982 Aug;44(3):621-31.

The utility of Hyman Rodman's theory of resources in cultural context for understanding decision-making patterns among spouses in intergenerationally linked **Puerto Rican** families in the United States is assessed using U.S. Census Data for the New York City area.   Significant differences found in assimilation between the parent's and child's generations support the hypothesis that the sociocultural norms of the parent generation, born and raised in Puerto Rico, reflect those of a modified patriarchal society, while the sociocultural norms of the child generation, born and raised in the U.S., reflect those of a transitional egalitarian society.   The theory of resources in cultural context leads to the expectation that level of assimilation acts as a contingency variable affecting the relationship between socioeconomic attributes and decision-making.   Findings support the expectation that husbands in the parent generation with higher socioeconomic achievements reflecting socialization to modern values had less power in decision-making, while husbands in the child generation with higher socioeconomic achievements representing power resources had greater power in decision-making.

67. Cromwell RE ; Ruiz RA. The myth of macho dominance in
decision-making within Mexican and Chicano families. **Hispanic
Journal of Behavioral Sciences.** 1979 Oct;1(4):355-73.

The myth concerning Hispanic family life which prevails in the
social science literature can best be summarized by abbreviated
quotations attributed to Alvirez and Bean.   The **Mexican** or
Chicano husband is a macho autocrat who rules as absolute head
of the family with full authority over the wife and children,
where all major decisions are his responsibility.   Domination by
husbands in marriage is logically consistent with their wives'.
submissiveness accompanied by passive acceptance of the future,
strong religious beliefs, and a tendency to reside in the temporal present.   The myth is also deeply embedded in the social
pathology model; differences between Hispanics and Anglos are
assumed to reflect negatively on Hispanics. The myth, it should
be noted, is seldom subjected to the scrutiny of empirical
inquiry. The review of four studies on both Mexican and Chicano
samples fails to support the notion of male dominance in marital
decision-making.   Refutation of the hypothesis of masculine
dominance in marital decision-making calls other components of
the myth into question.

68. *Darabi KF ; Namerow PB ; Philliber SG. The fertility-
related attitudes of Mexican Americans. Revised version of a
paper presented at the Annual Meeting of the Population Association of America, Pittsburgh, Pennsylvania. April 14-16, 1983.
(Unpublished) 16 p.

Four fertility related attitudes of **Mexican** Americans were compared with those of non-Hispanic blacks and whites.   The data
were from the cumulative General Social Surveys and include
pooled information from eight NORC personal interview studies
conducted from 1972-78 and in 1980 and 1982.   This cumulative
sample included 13,626 English speaking respondents aged 18
years or older.   Mexican Americans and whites had more liberal
attitudes toward the availability of contraceptive and sex information than did blacks, and Mexican Americans reported larger
ideal family sizes than did the other two groups.   In the multivariate analyses, after control for demographic and social differences was introduced, it appeared that ethnicity per se had
little to do with abortion attitudes or feelings about the
availability of sex and contraceptive information.   Relative to
blacks, both whites and Mexican Americans had more conservative
attitudes toward premarital sex.   Compared to whites, both
blacks and Mexican Americans expressed a desire for more children.   The findings suggest that stereotypes of Mexican Americans as generally more conservative than non-Hispanics on all
fertility-related attitudes are inaccurate.

69. *Davis SM ; Harris MB. Adolescents' questions about sex.
Journal of Adolescent Health Care. 1983 Dec;4(4):225-9.

Male and female adolescents from urban and rural areas were
given a chance to ask anonymous questions about sex.   These
questions were then used as the bases for subsequent presenta-
tions on sex education.   Subjects were 185 female and 103 male
students from two urban and three rural public schools, ranging
in age from 11 to 18 years.   There were 110 Anglos, 99 Hispanics, and 64 Native Americans.   Students were asked to indicate their sex, age and ethnicity.   The most popular categories
of questions were reproduction, sexuality, and contraception;

followed by anatomy, venereal disease, pregnancy, abortion, vocabulary, hygiene, and other diseases. Younger adolescents asked significantly more questions in most categories than older ones. Girls asked significantly more total questions and ones concerning pregnancy, contraception and anatomy than boys. Students attending rural schools asked more questions about venereal disease than those in urban schools, but no other main effects of urban/rural location were found. There were no differences between Hispanics and Anglos. A sample of questions asked by students is included in an appendix.

70. *Davis SM ; Harris MB. Sexual knowledge, sexual interests, and sources of sexual information of rural and urban adolescents from three cultures. **Adolescence**. 1982 Summer;17(66):471-92.

A total of 288 students aged 11 to 18 from five public schools in New Mexico were surveyed in order to determine if their sources of sexual information, sexual interests, and actual knowledge were related to their sex, age, urban or rural residence, and ethnicity. The ethnic breakdown was as follows: 39% were Anglo; 36% were Hispanic; and 24% were Native Americans. Female subjects were generally more knowledgeable than males about facts of maturation and reproduction, pregnancy, and contraception, as well as more interested than males in a number of sexual terms. Urban students indicated a greater familiarity than rural students with several of the terms. Anglos were generally the most knowledgeable, followed by Hispanics and Native Americans, with several ethnic differences in interests. Older students knew more facts and were more interested in pregnancy and birth control than younger students. Friends were the most common source of sexual information, followed by schools, books/magazines, and parents. Anglos, females, and students from rural areas received more information from their parents than males, Hispanics, Native Americans, and students from urban areas.

71. *Decker DL ; Caetano DF. Variations in natal knowledge among high school students. **Journal of School Health**. 1977 May; 47(5):286-8.

In developing health education programs it is essential to be aware of, and then take into account, the different levels of knowledge of the students the programs are designed to serve. This study was conducted to determine the differences in the level of natal knowledge in a high school sample in which there are large numbers of diverse racial and ethnic members. A questionnaire was distributed to 1,128 high school students: 43% were female and 57% were male; 66% were white, 19% black and 15% **Mexican** American; 32% were Protestant, 34% Catholic, 3% Jewish, 32% reported no religion, and .1% other. Whites had the largest proportion of high scores (i.e., 57% or more questionnaire items correct) with 36%, followed by blacks with 31%, and Mexican Americans 24%. In every case the females scored higher than the males. The low scores of Mexican Americans in this sample suggest that this group should be a target for the dissemination of natal knowledge.

72. *Edington E ; Hays L. Differences in family size and marriage age expectation and aspirations of Anglo, Mexican American and Native American rural youth in New Mexico. **Adolescence**. 1978;13:393-400.

A neglected area of family research is the study of marriage and procreation expectations and aspirations of youth. Questionnaires were given to 587 sophomore and senior students in 12 rural high schools in New Mexico during January and February of 1975.   Schools were selected to provide a representative cross-section of reference groups: Anglos, **Mexican** Americans, and Native Americans. Respondents were questioned relative to their marital and procreation aspirations and expectations.   Findings included: 1)   significant differences existed   between   ethnic groups in age expected and desired for marriage; 2) no differences existed between age groups for expected and aspired age of marriage or number of children; 3) a proportionately larger number of Native Americans were not future oriented in aspirations and expectations than Anglos and Mexican Americans. Significant differences also existed between ethnic groups in family size expectations and family size aspirations.

73.   *Eisen M ; Zellman GL. Factors predicting pregnancy resolution decision satisfaction of unmarried adolescents. **Journal of Genetic Psychology**. 1984 Dec;145(2d half):231-9.

Two hundred and ninety-nine premaritally pregnant Caucasian and **Mexican** American adolescents aged 13 to 19 who received pregnancy counseling, pregnancy termination, or prenatal services at a county clinic were reinterviewed six months after delivery or abortion to assess postdecision satisfaction.   More than 80% making each decision (i.e., abortion, single motherhood, marriage) said they would make the same decision again. There were no significant effects of decision alternative, ethnicity/ religion, or age on satisfaction.   Among aborters, four factors: positive preprocedure abortion opinion, more liberal attitudes towards abortion for others, consistent contraceptive use following abortion, and their mothers' higher educational attainment accounted for about 20% of the variance in satisfaction. Among single mothers, positive preprocedure attitude towards single motherhood and lack of attempts to attend school in the six months after delivery were associated in bivariate analysis with decision satisfaction.   Implications of these findings for adolescent pregnancy counseling are discussed.

74.   *Eisen M ; Zellman GL. Health belief model based changes in sexual knowledge, attitudes and behavior. Austin, Texas, University of Texas, Texas Population Research Center. 1984. (Texas Population Research Center Paper No. 6.021).

The evaluation of the Health Belief Model based educational intervention as a means of increasing adolescents' fertility control through abstinence or effective contraceptive usage is discussed.   One hundred and forty six Texas adolescents (55% Anglo, 21% black, 24% Hispanic) participated in the preintervention and postintervention phases of the program. Results of the intervention indicated modest, but statistically significant, changes in health belief perceptions, and substantial ones in sexuality and contraceptive knowledge.   The curriculum appears to be equally applicable to white, black and Hispanic participants with some exceptions (some health beliefs of Hispanics changed less than did those of other groups and males' knowledge increased less than did females' knowledge). There were modest, but statistically significant increases in reported contraceptive usage following the program. Limitations of the study are discussed.

75. Erickson PI ; Kaplan CP ; Scrimshaw SM. Contraceptive acceptability and desired family size among primiparous Mexican women in Los Angeles. Paper presented at the 113th Annual Meeting of the American Public Health Association, Washington, D.C. November 17-21, 1985.

This paper describes the level of contraceptive knowledge and acceptability for 518 **Mexican** American women in the Los Angeles area. These women were part of a study of births in Hispanic women funded by NICHD. Contraceptive knowledge and acceptability were measured by familiarity with 12 birth control methods, past use of birth control, and future intentions of contraception. The relationship between contraceptive acceptability and desired family size is explored. Also described is how acculturation, partner support and other demographic variables such as age and education affect both desired family size and contraceptive acceptability. The data show that these women are, in general, familiar with methods of birth control, and intend to use highly effective methods after the birth of their first child in order to space their children. These women wanted to wait an average of 3.2 years before having their next child and wanted an average of 1.9 more children after this birth. These women believed that their partners wanted an average of .87 more children than they themselves wanted. Implications for postpartum delivery of family planning services are explored.

76. Esparza R. The value of children among lower class Mexican, Mexican American and Anglo couples. Doctoral Dissertation, University of Michigan. 1977. DAI;38(3-B):1397.

Using the theoretical model of fertility behavior proposed by Hoffman and Hoffman, four cultural groups (**Mexican** Catholics, Mexican American Catholics, Anglo Catholics, and Anglo Protestants) were compared on values contributing to: the decision to have children or not, family size, and the preferred sex of children. Thirty couples in each of the four groups (total n=240) were selected from couples attending a community health clinic in Detroit, Michigan. A questionnaire was used to collect data on the value of children, the costs of and barriers to fertility, and family planning. The respondents valued children for reasons under the major Hoffman and Hoffman (1973) categories of primary group ties, stimulation, expansion of self, adult status and economic utility. Positive values differed across groups in the degree of importance attached to each value. Further differences were noted regarding attitudes concerning childlessness and one child families, value satisfactions, and values concerning life in general. In varying degrees, the groups expressed costs in terms of economic or emotional disadvantages. These particular costs were heavily influenced by social conditions in Detroit during 1975. Differences were observed in attitudes, methods, usage and decision-making regarding birth control.

77. Falk WW ; Falkowski CK ; Hansen GL. Further consideration of the fertility/work plans relationship. Paper of the Rural Sociological Society. (Unpublished) 1981.

The authors examined to what degree fertility attitudes and behaviors impact on labor force participation, utilizing data on female respondents from the National Longitudinal Study of the high school class of 1972. The analysis includes panel data with repeated measures on the key dependent variables (expanded to include fertility, labor force, marital, and educational plans) and a tri-ethnic comparison between whites, blacks, and **Mexican** Americans. The results are highly supportive of the work of Waite and Stolzenberg (1976), and Cramer (1980) in that labor force plans are found to be more important for fertility plans than is true of the reverse relationship. Marital and educational plans are of importance in understanding the more general case of the formation of life plans. In all cases, however, a life plan at one time is the best predictor of itself at a later point in time.

78. Farris BE ; Glenn ND. Fatalism and familism among Anglos and Mexican Americans in San Antonio. **Sociology and Social Research.** 1976;60:393-402.

Social scientists have often maintained that some of the characteristic values of **Mexican** Americans tend to hamper economic and social advancement, fatalism and familism being the values most often mentioned. The Mexican American data for this study were collected by the Wesley Youth Project for the UCLA Mexican American project, and the Anglo data come from a survey conducted in 1966 by the Wesley Youth Project in conjunction with the UCLA project. A comparison of the responses of Anglos and Mexican Americans to interview items designed to measure fatalism and familism shows a moderate ethnic difference in fatalism and a larger difference in familism. Controls for education largely remove the difference in fatalism, but at each educational level the Mexican Americans appear, as a whole, to have been distinctly more familistic than the Anglos. Since fatalism, rather than familism is emphasized in most cultural handicap explanations for the low socioeconomic status of Mexican Americans, the findings lend little support to those explanations.

79. *Fielder EP ; Becerra RM. The role of social support networks on Latino adolescent sexual attitudes and behavior. Paper presented at the 113th Annual Meeting of the American Public Health Association, Washington, D.C. November 17-21, 1985.

Traditionally, Latinos live in a close-knit, extended family network. Since the process of acculturation is believed to have somewhat eroded the traditional family structure, this family model is believed to best fit the unacculturated **Mexican** American family whose primary language is Spanish. Additionally, the influence of peers in the social network on attitudes and behavior has been documented for blacks and whites. Very little, however, is known about the role of family and peers with respect to Mexican American adolescent sexual attitudes and behavior. The aim of this paper is to assess the importance of peer and family networks on Mexican American adolescent sexual attitudes and behavior, focusing on the effects of various levels of acculturation and socioeconomic status. The data are based on a community survey of 1,000 adolescent females, aged 13 to 19 (700 Mexican Americans and 300 Anglo Americans). The sample was selected through multistage probability sampling techniques using 1980 Los Angeles County Census data.

80. *Fletcher PL. A comparison of adolescent sex role perceptions among male and female Anglo and Chicano ninth graders in southern New Mexico. Doctoral Dissertation. 1979. 88 p. DAI;40 (6-A):3083.

Adolescent sex role perceptions of male and female Anglo and Chicano (**Mexican**) ninth graders were investigated with a specially designed instrument, the Adolescent Duo-Ethnic Sex Role Perception Inventory. Twenty-three ninth grade classes containing Anglos and Chicanos of both sexes from 13 public schools in southern New Mexico were administered the measure. The inventory was divided into five subscales: traditional female role, traditional male role, education, career/leadership, and equality of opportunity and responsibility. Significant differences between the sexes were found for all subscales, and significant differences between the ethnic groups were found on four of five subscales. Chicanos and males were found to be significantly more traditional than Anglos and females, respectively.

81. *Gonzalez A. Sex roles of the traditional Mexican family: a comparison of Chicano and Anglo students' attitudes. **Journal of Cross-Cultural Psychology**. 1982 Sep;13(3):330-9.

This study examines the degree to which Chicano and Anglo students agree on sex roles as described in literature characterizing the traditional **Mexican** family. The subjects were 524 undergraduate students from California State University. The subjects were divided into four groups as follows: Chicano male (n=90), Chicano female (n=102), Anglo male (n=109), and Anglo female (n=154). A questionnaire was developed by reviewing the literature on the Mexican family and extracting statements about the ideal behavior for each of the sexes. Results of the questionnaire yielded significant differences for sex and ethnicity, with Chicano males agreeing more with stereotypic sex roles than Chicano females and Anglo males and females. The traditional Mexican family sex roles as described in the literature did not find support as an accurate representation of Chicano attitudes. In fact, the results indicate the opposite in general, with the exception of the rather neutral position of the Chicano male.

82. Gray SS. **A source book on child welfare: serving Chicano families and children.** Ann Arbor, Michigan, University of Michigan, School of Social Work. 1983.

This source book is intended as resource material for health and social workers who work with Chicano (**Mexican**) families. Each chapter includes references, abstracts, tables of contents, illustrative material and comments on relevant published books and articles. The areas covered are: families, cultural issues, delivery of services, education/training, and resource organizations. The section on families compiles resources that depict the Chicano family with an emphasis on human relationships and a strong sense of community that extends beyond the nuclear family. The section on cultural issues includes works on the historical experiences of the Chicano, beginning with Spanish colonization and extending to the migration to the United States. The last section identifies national organizations that provide a wide range of services for Chicano families and children.

83. Gray SS. **A source book on child welfare: serving Puerto Rican families and children.** Ann Arbor, Michigan, University of Michigan, School of Social Work. 1984.

This source book is intended as resource material for health and social workers who work with **Puerto Rican** families. Each chapter includes references, abstracts, tables of contents, illustrative material and comments on relevant published books and articles. The areas covered are: families, cultural issues, delivery of services, education/training, and resource organizations. The chapter on families covers Spanish colonial culture, slavery, economic development, the modern family, intermarriage, migration and family, and cultural values. The section on cultural issues includes the history of racism, and other historical experiences. The chapter on delivery of services deals with cultural sensitivity, family therapy and training of service providers.

84. Hanson RA. Household density, size of families and selected aspects of life quality of Mexican American families. Doctoral Dissertation, University of California. 1980. 185 p. DAI;41(6-A):2781.

The relationship between perceived quality of life and living locale, familism, family satisfaction, and other variables was examined in 101 Mexican American married couples with at least one child, living in a metropolitan or rural area. The predicted higher family satisfaction among males relative to females failed to reach significance, but the predicted higher satisfaction for rural families was confirmed. Family size and respondent age were unrelated to family satisfaction only for males. A consistent negative relationship was found between number of years married and reported satisfaction. Perceived quality of life was higher for the rural subjects, but was significant only for females. Generally, there was no relationship between quality of life and income or age, and the relationship to education was significant only for urban subjects. Relationships between family density and marital/family satisfaction were inconclusive. Overall, much of the stereotyping of Mexican Americans was not supported by results; males were as interested in the family as women; and the traditional dominance/submissive sex role pattern was not found.

85. Hawkes GR ; Taylor M. Power structure in Mexican and Mexican American farm labor families. **Journal of Marriage and the Family**. 1975 Nov;37(4):807-11.

An attempt is made to explain why a more egalitarian family power structure was found for Mexicans or Mexican Americans than was expected. Scientific and popular literature has stressed the dominant role of the male in these cultures. Familial power structure in Mexican and Mexican American farm labor families was explored by standardized interviews to determine if the commonly held view of husband dominance could be substantiated. As part of a national study of disadvantaged families, the authors, from 1971-73, studied family patterns of California migrant farm labor families. In 76 cases from California state operated family migrant labor camps, egalitarianism was by far the most common mode in both decision-making and action taking. The traditional forces of change, acculturation, and urbanization were not found to be responsible for results found in this particular investigation. Dominance/submission patterns are much less universal than previously assumed, or never existed but were an ideal, or are undergoing radical change.

86. Hoffman LW ; Manis JD. The value of children in the United States: a new approach to the study of fertility. **Journal of Marriage and the Family**. 1979 Aug;41(3):583-96.

A study of national sample data regarding attitudes toward
raising children and fertility found positively related satisfactions were less common in America, but cited more by subgroups with higher fertility desires.   Primary group ties and
affection was the advantage most cited in the United States.
Women cited this value more often than men.   Less educated men
and women scored higher in this category.   Black fathers were
the exception in that they rated stimulation and fun equally as
high as primary group ties and affection.   Less educated black
mothers rated primary group ties and affection highest (73%),
followed by black fathers (70%), Hispanic mothers (69%), less
educated white mothers (66%), and college educated white mothers
(64%).   The sampling, field work, and coding were conducted by
the Institute for Social Research at the University of Michigan.
The sample consisted of 1,569 married women under age 40 and 456
of their husbands.   The interview was given at the respondents'
home and took one hour and 20 minutes.

87. Hoppe SK ; Heller PL. Alienation, familism and the utilization of health services by Mexican Americans. **Journal of Health
and Social Behavior**. 1975 Sep;16(3):304-14.

This study examines the influence of familism and occupational
stability on alienation and health care utilization among lower
class **Mexican** Americans.   The data used in this paper were collected by interviews with 197 Mexican American women in San
Antonio, Texas, during the summer of 1972.   It was found that
familism and occupational stability were positively related to
timing of prenatal care, but negatively related to consulting a
physician when ill.   Powerlessness was negatively related to
timing of prenatal care and positively related to consulting
when ill.   The results suggest it is important to distinguish
preventive and curative components of health care behavior in
measures of utilization.   The observed associations between
familism, occupational stability, powerlessness, and curative
health behavior are undoubtedly related to issues of the economic accessibility of care.   In addition, the role of familism
should be considered in the complex relationship between alienation and health care utilization.

88. Horowitz R. **Honor and the American dream: culture and
identity in a Chicano community**. New Brunswick, New Jersey, Rut-
gers University Press. 1983.

This anthropological report of a year's field work in a Chicano
(**Mexican**) community in Chicago focuses upon young people and the
process of growing up.   Several chapters describe attitudes and
norms related to dating, preservation of virginity, sex role
attitudes, traditional family values and adolescent childbearing.   In the chapter on The Expanded Family and Family Honor,
the author describes a cotillion or "quinceanera" (fifteenth
birthday party) which symbolizes much of what is valued in the
Chicano family: the close, interdependent family network and the
family's success in finances; in containing the sexual activities of the daughter so that she not only remains a virgin, but
is perceived as such; and in following the proper forms of
social interaction.   Unmarried women know about birth control,
but often do not use it because it would be an explicit indica-
tion of her intention to engage in sexual intercourse.   She
cannot explain such action as a moment of passion, the culturally acceptable account.   Moreover, birth control is perceived
as allowing a woman to engage in sex whenever and with whomever

she pleases, the archetypal instance of unbounded sexuality. Her passion need not be controlled. She is also explicitly negating the importance of motherhood. Thus the use of birth control is thought to provide consummate evidence of an unmarried woman's impurity.

89. Hotvedt ME. Family planning among Mexican Americans of South Texas. Doctoral Dissertation, Indiana University. 1976. 295 p. DAI;37(4-A):2277.

An ethnograph of a Texas Chicano community was presented emphasizing social roles and attitudes of women on the subject of birth control in an historical framework. Participant observation within the community, open ended interviews, and written questionnaires were used to explore motivational factors for the women's acceptance or rejection of birth control usage and family planning philosophy. Findings indicated a large degree of intracommunity acceptance of birth control use for married couples, with minimal concern for the Roman Catholic Church's stand on birth control, although most informants considered themselves active Catholics. Individuals most influential in birth control decisions were spouses and close kinswomen, and factors most influential included economics, social class, concern for the marital relationship, material and spiritual well being of children, and career advancement. An area of conflict was identified in premarital couples, where change was seen resulting from contact with Anglo values expressed in school expectations, urban living, wage labor, and media images.

90. Klitz SI. Cross-cultural communication: the Hispanic community of Connecticut. Storrs, Connecticut, University of Connecticut. 1980. 65 p.

This paper includes a general discussion and definition of several traditional Hispanic values. The quality of machismo is examined. Men are given a great deal of latitude in marriage, and extramarital affairs are indicators of the degree of masculinity. Sex roles are defined early in life. Promiscuity in boys is indulgently chuckled at, secretly admired. Girls, on the other hand, are taught that chastity is the ultimate objective of their training. There are two types of marriage which are acknowledged in the **Puerto Rican** community: the consensual union and the official union. The consensual union is usually taken more seriously by the wife, who considers herself married when she gives herself to her husband. From the husband's point of view, however, consensual marriage is not as binding as legal marriage. The traditional roles of the Hispanic male and female are rapidly being altered by contact with mainlanders. Increased awareness of female sexuality, the mobilization of women as part of the work force, and the availability of educational opportunities for women are influencing the values of the old world.

91. Kranau EJ ; Green V ; Valencia-Weber G. Acculturation and the Hispanic woman: attitudes toward women, sex role attribution, sex role behavior, and demographics. **Hispanic Journal of Behavioral Science.** 1982 Mar;4(1):21-40.

The study investigates the relationship of acculturation to the variables of attitudes toward women, sex role attribution, sex role behaviors, and demographics in Hispanic women. First, 60 **Mexican** American, **Puerto Rican, Cuban, Peruvian,** and **Bolivian** women were investigated to determine if they could be placed on a continuum of acculturation.   Second, the relationship between different levels of acculturation and the above variables was investigated.   Last, the predictive power of these variables to acculturation level was determined through multiple regression techniques.   The sample drawn did not significantly differ from the original population used in acculturation research by Olmedo, Martinez, and Martinez, indicating that the Mexican American woman can be placed on a continuum of acculturation regardless of age or geographical location.   Greater acculturation was positively correlated with more liberal attitudes toward women, single status, more education, and younger age. Greater acculturation was negatively correlated with more feminine household behaviors.   The best subset of predictors of acculturation was found to be education and self-attribution of feminine and masculine sex role characteristics.

92. *Leibowitz A ; Eisen M ; Chow W. An economic model of teenage pregnancy decision-making. **Demography**. 1986 Feb;23(1): 67-77.

Data for the analysis were derived from a previous study of 386 pregnant adolescents, aged 13 to 19, who used either the pre-natal or termination services of health care providers in Ventura County, California between 1972-74.   Teenage fertility decisions are frequently considered to be irrational or emotionally based.   However, a closer examination of pregnancy trends among teenagers reveals that they make rational assessments of the costs and benefits of their fertility options.   Therefore, the use of an economic model for analyzing their decisions was deemed appropriate.   It was hypothesized that the availability of welfare increases the probability that an unmarried pregnant teenager will choose to be an unmarried mother rather than to terminate the pregnancy or to marry.   Respondents were categorized as either **Mexican** Americans, non-Catholic and non-Mexican American, or Catholic and non-Mexican American.   The dependent variable was the pregnancy decision.   Independent variables included: value of time variables, public assistance and self-support variables, and ethnic and religious variables.   The findings supported the hypothesis.   Mexican Americans were more likely to choose to marry or to be a single mother than to terminate their pregnancies.

93. Linn MW ; Carmichael JS ; Klitenick P ; Webb N ; Gurel L. Fertility-related attitudes of minority mothers with large and small families. **Journal of Applied Social Psychology**. 1978 Jan/ Mar;8(1):1-14.

The authors examined the relationship between certain attitudes and levels of fertility in five cultural groups: blacks, **Cubans**, American Indians, migrant Chicanos (**Mexicans**), and white Protestants.   In general, mothers in large families wanted fewer children than they had.   The trend was reversed in the migrant group where small family mothers were more negative toward birth control.   Among the Chicanos, the deviant pattern was a small family.   In this group the direction of attitudes was reversed related to fertility.   It was the small and not the large family mothers who were more negative toward birth control.   Although Cubans said they wanted more children, and had more favorable attitudes toward family, pregnancy, and parent, their overall fertility was slightly lower than white Protestants.   Likewise, although their attitudes toward abortion were more negative than the other subcultures, over twice as many Cubans had had abortions than any other group. Chicanos said they wanted, and they had, the largest number of children; the large family mothers averaged 7.3.   Large family Cuban and white mothers averaged only 5.8 and 5.9 children, but large family white mothers wanted fewer children and Cuban mothers about what they had.

94. Marin G ; Marin BV ; Padilla AM. The meaning of children for Hispanic women. Los Angeles, California, University of California, Spanish Speaking Mental Health Research Center. (Unpublished) 1981. 15 p.

A random sample of 100 Hispanic women waiting to receive birth control services at a low cost community health center in East Los Angeles were interviewed to learn more about the fertility behavior, attitudes toward family size, and contraceptive use of barrio Hispanic women.   The respondents were: young (averaging 27 years old), poorly educated (averaging 7.43 years of schooling), of low socioeconomic status ($666 average monthly household income), married (66%), mostly of **Mexican** origin (80%), and recent immigrants (85% being first generation Hispanics, i.e., born in Latin America). Results indicated the younger the women at the birth of their first child, the more children they had and desired.   Those with fewer years of schooling had larger families.   The best predictor of a woman's desired family size was her perception of her spouse's desired family size.   Being born in Latin America was positively associated with larger desired family size.   The value placed on children by these Hispanic women and their husbands appeared to be a major factor in their higher fertility rate, a value formed by their culture, yet subject to acculturative influences.

95. Miller MV. Variations in Mexican American family life: a review synthesis of empirical research. **Aztlan.** 1978;9:209-31.

Mexican American families generally have been conceptualized, both popularly and academically, as traditional units characterized by extreme familism, and rigid age and sex role differentiation.   These presumed traits have frequently been used to account for the persistence of poverty, the lack of significant upward economic mobility and other alleged social pathologies of this population.   Accordingly, acculturation to the prevailing United States middle class family model has been suggested as the broad panacea for these problems.   After a critique of the acculturation model as theory and ideology, the prevailing idea of the traditional Mexican American family is assessed through an extensive review of relevant contemporary research.   Findings suggest that: 1) exaggerated familism is not a predominant feature of urban Mexican American life, regardless of region or socioeconomic level; 2) family roles are variable and dynamic, influenced by immediate economic circumstances confronting families; 3) the magnitude and impact of kinship arrangements varies significantly by place of residence and nativity; and 4) interethnic marriage is an increasing phenomenon, although still sensitive to the nature of local interethnic relations.

96. Mirande A. The Chicano family: a reanalysis of conflicting views. **Journal of Marriage and the Family.** 1977 Nov;39(4):747-56.

Two conflicting views of the **Mexican** American (Chicano) family are examined.   The traditional social science view depicts a rigid, male-dominated, authoritarian structure that breeds passivity and dependence. A more sympathetic perspective views the family as a warm, nurturing, and supportive environment which gives its members a strong sense of security. Although the second view dispels many erroneous, negative stereotypes about the Chicano family, it generates a positive set of stereotypes. After reevaluating these earlier perspectives, a new, more objective and viable view of the Chicano family is offered. Probably the most significant characteristic of the Chicano family is its strong emphasis on familism. While the impact of the family may have been eroded somewhat by urbanization and acculturation, it is still a central institution for the individual. The familistic orientation of Chicanos is such that relatives are frequently included as friends. Both pejorative and positive accounts of the Chicano family see the male as the ultimate and unquestioned authority in the family. Although the mother has been depicted as a lowly and insignificant figure, she is extremely important in intrafamily relationships.

97. *Mirande A. A reinterpretation of male dominance in the Chicano family. **Family Coordinator**. 1979 Oct;28(4):473-9.

A review of recent research studies suggests that the dominant pattern of decision-making and action taking in the Chicano (**Mexican**) family is not male-dominated and authoritarian, but egalitarian. Sex role segregation is rare. Husband and wife share not only in decisions, but in household tasks and child care. Sharp sex role segregation appears to be the exception rather than the rule among Chicano couples. In addition to theoretical and methodological implications, this new view of the Chicano family has significant implications both for the formulation of public policy and family counseling. A redefinition of machismo and the male role within the family is a critical first step in this process, since male dominance is assumed to be not only the cornerstone of the culture, but the source of much of the pathology found within the family and the Chicano community.

98. Mitchell JO. Minority attitudes toward contraception. **Journal of Reproductive Medicine**. 1974 Dec;13(6):212-5.

The training division of the Los Angeles Regional Family Planning Council conducted a seminar for minority members to discover attitudes toward birth control. Indian Americans, **Mexican** Americans, Asian Americans, and black Americans participated. Some fears and misunderstandings relative to birth control were voiced. The timidity of recent Chinese immigrants was mentioned. Male reluctance to use birth control out of a sense of machismo was mentioned in relation to blacks and Mexican Americans. The conclusion was that when birth control methods are adequately explained women of all ethnic groups are willing to use them. To allay fears, suspicions, and concerns, family planning should be presented to minority communities as a health service and not a social service. Family planning clinics would be more accepted in these communities if they expanded their work into other health areas.

99. *Moerk E. The acculturation of the Mexican American minority to the Anglo American society in the United States. **Journal of Human Relations**. 1972;20(3):317-25.

Epochal changes in the values and aspirations of **Mexican** American preadolescents and adolescents were compared with those of

other minority group and Anglo American youth.   In 1967 and
1970, a questionnaire was presented to 446 subjects of Anglo,
Mexican American, and black descent.   Educational and occupational aspirations, and expectations regarding future incomes
and the purchase of material goods were primarily explored in
1967.   Significant differences were generally found between
ethnic groups, with the Mexican American subjects having the
lowest aspirations.   Three years later the differences had
vanished or become so small as to be insignificant.   A sudden
increase in aspirations of the Mexican Americans was the cause,
and was accompanied by other acculturation processes.   In regard
to ideal family size, age at marriage, and acceptance of birth
control methods, Mexican American subjects had also approached
the standards of the larger American society.   Quick changes of
values and attitudes can be wrought even in populations from
lower social classes which are loyal to their traditional culture and religion, if the younger generation and strong ethnic
organizations are the carriers of these changes.

100. *Montes JM. Developmental dimensions of attitudes and
values related to judgments about an ideal family. Doctoral Dissertation, Ohio State University. 1976. 114 p. DAI;37(5-B):2516.

Attitudes and values which relate to the desirability of having
children, individual's responses to various dimensions of family
planning, and the presence of developmental trends with respect
to the processes involved in family planning were studied in
ninth through twelfth grade adolescents and young married people
without children.   Ninety-eight percent of the subjects were of
Mexican American descent.   Tentative conclusions were that there
were strong developmental trends in attitudes and values and
that with increasing psychological maturity: 1) both males and
females become more realistic and less romantic about the responsibilities involved in having children;   2) both become less
willing to accept social/cultural stereotypical considerations
as good sufficient reasons for having children;   3) both become
less willing to accept the idea that having children insures a
happier or more stable marital relationship;   4) both become more
rejecting of the proposition that having children should be a
privilege reserved for more intelligent and gifted adults;   5)
both remain consistently undecided about the advantages or disadvantages of interracial marriages;   6) there are several differential trends among males and females with respect to family
planning and the siring and bearing of children.

101. *Moss N ; Barnett C ; Alvarez A. Response to adolescent
pregnancy in Mexican American and Anglo families.   Paper presented at the American Public Health Association Annual Meeting,
Montreal, Canada. (Unpublished) 1982. 12 p.

The data presented are from a hypothesis generating study of
adolescent pregnancy in San Jose.   The purpose of the study was
to develop a model of health related risk taking behavior during
pregnancy.   Half of the 40 teenagers under 18 interviewed in the
qualitative study were **Mexican** American, half were Anglo.   About
62% of the survey respondents were Mexican American, 25% were
Anglo.   Despite differences, families in both ethnic groups were
overwhelmingly poor and undereducated.   About half of the adolescents in the study were in intact marriages at the time of the
pregnancy.   Before pregnancy three-fourths of the Anglos, but
only half the Chicanas, were living with parents.   They lived
with partners, relatives, in foster homes, or in frequent tran-

sition between situations.   While Anglo and Chicano parents are
equally likely to provide financial help, the pregnant Chicana
and her partner are more likely to be given shelter during the
pregnancy by her family than by his. The Mexican American culture places strong emphasis on family ties, on the obligations
of parents to children, and the duties of children to parents.
In Chicana culture, there are strong bonds between mothers and
daughters, and between females in general.

102. *Mott FL ; Mott SH. Attitude consistency among American
youth. Columbus, Ohio, Ohio State University, Center for Human
Resource Research. 1982. 28 p.

Attitudes of youth aged 14 to 21 toward fertility expectations
and women's roles are examined for consistency (e.g., whether
high career expectations are correlated with a desire for fewer
children).   Approximately 12,000 white, black, and Hispanic
youth rated their attitudes toward statements that a woman's
place is in the home, employment of wives leads to juvenile
delinquency, employment of both parents is an economic necessity, men should share housework, and women are happier when
they stay at home.   Results indicated that most youth tend to
have non-traditional views on the role of women, although Hispanic youth are more likely than their black and white counterparts to believe that a woman's place is in the home. Young men
and women who expect to complete more education have less traditional views.   Of the three ethnic groups, only black youth do
not show congruence between attitudes toward women's roles and
fertility expectations.   Evidence also suggests that as they
grow older, more youth view home and non-home roles as potentially conflicting. Females show greater consistency than males
between fertility expectations and their view of women's role.

103. *Mott FL ; Mott SH. Prospective life style congruence
among ·American adolescents: variations in the association between fertility expectations and ideas regarding women's roles.
Social Forces. 1984 Sep;63(1):184-208.

This study uses data from the National Longitudinal Survey of
Labor Market Experience of Youth for a representative sample of
about 12,000 American youth, who where 14 to 21 years of age in
1979, to examine the extent of congruence between the attitudes
of young men and women about the appropriate roles for women and
their own fertility expectations.   Hispanic men and women have,
on average, more traditional views than their white and black
counterparts.   This tendency reflects their lesser assimilation
into the larger society.   In almost all cases, the foreign born
youth (both men and women) have more traditional values than the
native born youth.   Indeed, in a number of instances, the attitudes of the native born Hispanic youth do not differ markedly
from those of all American youth.   Attitudes for native born
Hispanic youth that still differ from those of other American
youth fall between attitudes of the foreign born Hispanic youth
and the white group.   Unlike black and white youth, Hispanic
youth follow the traditional pattern of inverse association
between educational and fertility expectations, perhaps reflecting their different stage·in the assimilation process.

104. Murillo-Rhode I. Family life among mainland Puerto Ricans
in New York City slums. **Perspectives in Psychiatric Care.**
1976;14(4):174-9.

Puerto Rican families who migrated to New York City in the 1950s are threatened by a system of impersonal relationships and norms which are at odds with their traditional values.   Puerto Rican families have a tendency to have many children.   A woman must have a child as soon as possible after marriage to show the community and her husband that she is fecund, and may be forbidden by her husband to use contraceptives.   Many of the women resort to sterilization.   Common-law marriages are found frequently among the lower socioeconomic families.   Mainland Puerto Rican families find problems trying to raise girls as virgins and boys with sexual freedom.   The daughters want to adopt the dominant pattern of mainland society.   The research is based on personal experience of the author as a nurse, educator and family therapist in East Harlem from 1964 to 1969.

105. *Namerow PB ; Philliber SG. Attitudes toward sex education among black, Hispanic and white inner city residents. **International Quarterly of Community Health Education.** 1982/1983;3(3): 291-9.

Telephone survey data gathered from residents of a New York City neighborhood indicate that Hispanics are significantly less likely to approve of sex education for adolescents than either blacks or whites.   Hispanics also perceive the appropriate ages for sex education to be older, and are more conservative about the topics and places for sex education than are the other ethnic groups. In terms of specific topics to be included in any sex education program, Hispanics are less likely than blacks or whites to approve of premarital sexuality, or of abortion as topics for discussion.   These differences remain after controls are introduced for sex, age, religion, education, number of children in the household, family income, or perception of teenage pregnancy as a problem.   Age and education, however, are also important predictors of attitudes toward sex education.   It seems clear from these findings that planning for sex education programs should not simply focus on the needs of minority populations.   The many attitudinal differences in this sample between the Hispanic and black minority groups clearly support the need to tailor programs to specific minorities.

106. *Pippin MU. An investigation of the self-reported problems of Mexican, Mexican American and Anglo American adolescents. Doctoral Dissertation, University of the Pacific. 1980. 203 p. DAI;41(4-A):1458.

Differences in problems reported by **Mexican**, Mexican American, and Anglo American adolescents of both sexes were examined and the influence of ethnicity, sex, and socioeconomic status of the differences studied.   Differences were found among all three groups and both sexes.   In all instances, however, the sex differences appeared to be a function of the differences between the Mexican genders.   When Mexican Americans and Anglo Americans were compared, statistical differences were found cross-culturally regardless of social class.   It is suggested that the Mexican Americans are a culturally definable entity.

107. *Ramirez M 3rd.   Identification with Mexican family values and authoritarianism in Mexican Americans. **Journal of Social Psychology.** 1967 Oct;73(1):3-11.

In this study it was hypothesized that **Mexican** American college students would score higher than Anglo Americans on a family

attitude F scale that reflected the values of the Mexican family, because their family milieu is very much like that of the
high authoritarians. The results indicate that the Mexican
American subjects made significantly higher scores than the
Anglo Americans on both the F scale and the Mexican Family
Attitude Scales. The Mexican American females made higher
scores on both scales than did any of the other three culture/
sex subgroups. The results indicate that young, middle class
Mexican Americans adhere to standards of conformity and authoritarian submission, indicating a need to maintain the status quo
and certainly to refrain from opposing it. Comparison of the
family attitude pattern of the Mexican Americans with that of
Mexicans and **Puerto Ricans** reveals that the Mexican American
value system shows signs of Americanization in the form of a
decrease in the authority of the male. The Mexican family
values on which the Mexican Americans expressed more agreement
than disagreement were those of conformity, strict child rearing, and authoritarian submission.

108. Roper BS ; Heath LL ; King CD. Racial consciousness: a new
guise for traditionalism? **Sociology** and **Social Research.** 1978
Apr;62(3):430-47.

This is a study to ascertain if minority groups' reproductive
attitudes and practices are changing. The data were collected
in a questionnaire administered to a tri-ethnic sample of 120
working class **Mexican** Americans, blacks, and whites in a west
Texas city selected by a disproportionately stratified systema-
tic sampling method. The survey found only limited evidence
linking racial consciousness to fertility differences, and the
observed association could be interpreted as based more on
traditional values than on a new, radical awareness. Traditionalism, the other factor, was found to be associated significantly with attitudes toward fertility and birth control. This
significance varied noticeably by age and minority group. The
results indicate that racial and ethnic awareness may pose
barriers to family planning and birth control programs. Thus,
as traditionalism is lost, it may be replaced by new attitudes
of racial consciousness, which will still emphasize high fertility.

109. *Rosenhouse-Persson S ; Sabagh G. Attitudes toward abortion among Catholic Mexican American women: the effects of
religiosity and education. **Demography.** 1983 Feb;20(1):87-98.

Catholic and non-Catholic attitudes toward abortion have not
been converging. This study suggests that this may be due to an
interaction between religiosity and education. In a sample of
Catholic **Mexican** American women in Los Angeles County, the
authors found that among respondents brought up in Mexico,
education had a liberalizing effect on their attitudes. With
the exception of the most devout, the same trend was observed
among respondents reared in the United States. Among the most
religious group, however, education had the opposite effect,
suggesting that convergence will be delayed. Data for the study
are from interviews with 1,129 Mexican American women aged 15 to
44 during a complex area probability sample of Los Angeles
households in 1973. Only women married to Mexican American men
are included in the sample due to cost limitations. It is suggested that the most educated, most religious group may fail to
adopt more liberal attitudes because higher education exposes
them to information on their church's specific stand on abor-

tion, on the controversy on the definition of when life begins,
and on exactly how the various birth control methods work.

110. Rothman J ; Gant LM ; Hnat SA. Mexican American family
culture. **Social Service Review.** 1985 Jun;59(2):197-215.

This article addresses the insufficient response of social work
practice and service delivery to racial and ethnic minorities.
A research based method is presented for identifying family cultural characteristics of the **Mexican** American ethnic group and
for designing intervention strategies.   Some of the limitations
of this method are indicated, as well as the necessity of field
intervention hypotheses in realistic practice settings.   Familism is perhaps the single most striking and consistent feature
of Chicano culture noted in the literature.   Studies have
indicated that Mexican Americans are more firmly rooted in the
family as a source of identification than either blacks or
Anglos, regardless of socioeconomic status or geographic locale
(i.e., urban/rural, or state of residence). However, it should
be noted that within the context of the traditional nuclear
patriarchy, Mexican American families are not structurally distinguishable from any other ethnic group with a similar family
orientation.   Chicano familism seems to be distinguishable by
its degree of family cohesiveness and by its extended definition
of family membership.

111. *Sabagh G. Fertility expectations and behavior among
Mexican Americans in Los Angeles: 1973-1982. **Social Science
Quarterly.** 1984 Jun;65(2):594-608.

The relationship between fertility expectations and behavior
among **Mexican** Americans in Los Angeles, California is explored.
The data are from a 1982 follow-up survey that included 70% of a
sample of 1,129 married Mexican American women originally surveyed in 1973.   As compared to the 1975 follow-up of the National Fertility Study, these women have a higher aggregate and
individual inconsistency between fertility expectations and
behavior.   Expectations were more predictive of the behavior of
women reared in the United States than those reared in Mexico.
Except for duration of marriage, these expectations had more
predictive power than a number of demographic and socioeconomic
variables.

112. *Salazar D. A cross-cultural analysis of the Chicano and
Anglo undergraduates' perceptions of sex role characteristics:
masculine, feminine, androgynous, and undifferentiated. Doctoral
Dissertation, Washington State University. 1979. 74 p. DAI;40(4-
A):1940.

To determine suitability of project awareness materials for
Chicano (**Mexican**) participants in sex role stereotyping work-
shops, Chicano and Anglo undergraduate perceptions of sex role
characteristics were examined using the Bem Sex Role Inventory
(BSRI). No significant differences were found between Anglo and
Chicano self-description among the four BSRI categories (masculine, feminine, androgynous, and undifferentiated). There were,
however, differences between Anglo and Chicano males and Anglo
and Chicano females with regard to specific adjectives in the
BSRI. On the basis of findings, it is concluded that, in general, project awareness materials are suitable for Chicano students at Washington State University.   Additional activities
are recommended to account for those few adjectives showing

differences between Chicano and Anglo groups. Further, the single cluster found for Anglo males corroborates the literature that challenges the desirability of the dominant society view of traditional masculinity. It is suggested that the concept of androgyny may be viewed as a more desirable alternative than sex role polarization implicit in traditional concepts of masculinity and femininity.

113. *Sanchez RB. Testimony at a hearing before the Subcommittee of the Committee on Education and Labor, Washington, D.C. July 24, 1978. House of Representatives, Ninety-fifth Congress, Second Session on H.R. 12146.

Text of a statement by Rodolfo B. Sanchez, the National Executive Director of the National Coalition of Hispanic Mental Health and Human Services Organizations (COSSMHO), concerning the Adolescent Health, Services, and Pregnancy Prevention and Care Act of 1978.   COSSMHO works to address the health, mental health, drug and alcohol abuse, and related human service needs of **Mexican** American, **Puerto Rican, Cuban,** and Latino communities throughout this country. A COSSMHO membership survey indicated that many Hispanics are deeply concerned about the increasing number of pregnant teenagers, the overall rise in premarital sexual activity, the intergenerational conflicts that may erupt as a result of adolescent pregnancy, and the dubious future prospects that may confront teenage parents and their children. The survey also revealed that for Hispanics, unlike many other communities in the nation, the problem and its solution call for not only better coordinated resources, but also more actual resources, and further require the application of these resources through projects and programs that acknowledge, respect, and strengthen the bilingual/bicultural context of Hispanic youth and their families.

114. *Santa Clara County Health Department. Natural family planning needs assessment questionnaire for Santa Clara County women of childbearing years. Santa Clara, California. (Unpublished) 1979. 17 p.

A questionnaire was distributed by family planning agencies, colleges, doctors, individuals, and other sources in January and February 1977 to determine if a need exists for teaching natural family planning to women of childbearing years in Santa Clara County, California and to learn if there is a need for teaching natural family planning (NFP) methods to medical, professional, and family personnel.   This report contains the overall percentages of all the returned women's questionnaires, including the questionnaires of 55 Spanish speaking women.   The symptothermal method and the Billings ovulation method were not known or understood by a large number of medical and professional personnel.   An overall comparison seems to indicate that women of childbearing years in Santa Clara County have a high interest in learning and using natural methods for family planning, whereas the interest on the part of medical and professional persons seems to be much lower concerning NFP methods and their practical usefulness to their clientele.   Both sectors seem to desire more education, research in use-effectiveness, and overall future usefulness of NFP methods.

115. *Sorenson AM. Fertility expectations and ethnic identity among -Mexican American adolescents: an expression of cultural ideals. **Sociological Perspectives.** 1985 Jul;28(3):339-60.

Survey data from Arizona secondary schools were used to test the
applicability of structural and minority status hypotheses to
the differential fertility expectations of **Mexican** American and
Anglo adolescents.   Analyses of the number of children expected
by these respondents and their implied parity progression ratios
indicate that indices of acculturation are more important in
explaining expected fertility than are measures of parental
socioeconomic status or respondent's expected status.   Among
Mexican American respondents, language spoken at home, nativity
of the respondent and his or her father, and residence are
associated with expected fertility.   These indices of acculturation retain their importance even when father's education, father's occupation and number of siblings are introduced.

116. Staples R. The Mexican American family: its modification
over time and space. **Phylon.** 1971 Summer;32(2):179-92.

A study of **Mexican** American marriage and family patterns,
changes resulting from Mexican Americans' transition from the
agrarian setting of Mexico to the urban, industrialized milieu
of the United States.   Interpretations and conclusions made are
based upon data gathered through two research techniques: a
review of the literature, and secondary data consisting of
interview documents with Mexican American clients of the author.
It is concluded that Mexican American family patterns are extremely variable and reflect the type of environment, the social
class membership and their adaptation to the changing forms of
American society.   Rural Mexican Americans are closest to the
extended family pattern.   Mexican Americans in the urban areas,
who have taken on the values of the Anglo American culture, have
more of a nuclear family pattern.   As the amount of assimilation
into the mores of the dominant society increases, the family
concept tends to narrow, with aunts, uncles, and cousins becoming less important.   The acculturation of the Mexican American
is a process that can be significantly facilitated or impeded by
their family structure and dynamics.

117. Staples R ; Mirande A. Racial and cultural variations
among American families: a decennial review of the literature on
minority families. **Journal of Marriage and the Family.** 1980;42
(4):887-903.

An assessment of the literature of the 1970s on Asian American,
black, Chicano (**Mexican**), and Native American families is presented.   Prior to 1970, minority families were subject to
negative stereotypes which were not empirically supported.   In
the case of blacks and Chicanos, the family literature of the
1970s represented an improvement because it depicted the positive aspects of their family life.   While black scholars faced
the task of refuting the myth of the matriarchy, Chicanos had to
deal with machismo and the issue of male dominance.   There
emerged, then, a sympathetic or revisionist view of the Chicano
family.   Theory and research on Asian and Native American families remained too limited to make any generalizations about
their family life styles.   The insider/outsider perspective
continues to be a source of controversy in the study of minority
families.   Future research needs to focus on the minority family
unit as an autonomous system with its own norms, rather than
comparing it to or contrasting it with the majority culture
using white, middle class standards.

118. *Staton RD. A comparison of Mexican and Mexican American

families. **The Family Coordinator.** 1972 Jul;21(3):325-30.

An attempt was made to ascertain some of the major features of the **Mexican** family which have been retained by the Mexican American family within the United States. Available literature which comment on the family systems was surveyed. Sufficient information for comparisons was found concerning male/female relationships, family organization, courtship and marriage, husband/wife relationships, and parent/child relationships. Masculine superiority, father dominance, and emphasis on submission and obedience to the authority of the father have been maintained by the Mexican American family. Present literature largely presents only a generalized view of both families. Many variables such as religion, social class, language, education, physical and social mobility, acculturation, and assimilation are not appropriately considered in the case of the Mexican American family. Therefore, empirical research which considers such factors must be undertaken before a true description and understanding of the Mexican American family can be obtained.

119. *Tamez EG. Familism, machismo and child rearing practices among Mexican Americans. **Journal of Psychosocial Nursing and Mental Health Services.** 1981 Sep;19(9):21-5.

Fertility is 50% higher in **Mexican** Americans than in any other ethnic group. Income levels are inordinately low. Fifty-two percent of all Mexican Americans do not finish high school. Paz and Remos described the Mexican in terms of Adler's inferiority model. Murillo stated that to an individual, the family (whether nuclear or extended), is the center of life, providing emotional and material security. Familism was seen as a deterrant to utilization of health care services, although some studies claim opposing views. Familism and occupational stability related positively to seeking medical care when ill. Hayden believed that supreme male dominance, individualism, pride, wife beating, aversion to contraceptives, and other characteristics were attributable to machismo. Role differentiation is taught implicitly and explicitly from infancy. Studies on the psychological differences between the sexes indicated that females were oppressed and had lower self-esteem than males. Eighteen to 24 year old Mexican Americans are becoming less insistent upon strict separation of sex roles and are beginning to reject the traditional Mexican notion of masculine superiority. Machismo is the underlying cause of family conflicts.

120. Tharp RG ; Meadow A ; Lennhoff S ; Satterfield D. Changes in marriage roles accompanying the acculturation of the Mexican American wife. **Journal of Marriage and the Family.** 1968 Aug;30(3):404-12.

The processes of acculturation as they affect marriage roles are examined in the **Mexican** American wife population of the United States southwest. Two groups, representing more and less acculturated populations, but roughly equivalent in age, are compared. A combination of area and cluster sampling techniques were employed, using home interview methods. Item responses were analyzed for group differences. Hypotheses were generally confirmed: during acculturation, marriage roles change toward a more egalitarian/companionate pattern or, in Rainwater's terms, from a segregated to a joint conjugal role pattern. Rainwater and Handel have illustrated for lower class families that changes in the prosperity level and the modern mobility of the family have led to the same kinds of conjugal and family role changes as was discovered between their two differently acculturated groups. With increasing socioeconomic status and position, the organization of conjugal roles changes from segregated to joint role relationship patterns. The results do not clarify whether the marriage roles of the Mexican American are primarily determined by socioeconomics or by the Mexican folk tradition. Such analyses will require comparative study of many cultures.

121. Tienda M. Familism and structural assimilation of Mexican immigrants in the United States. **International Migration Review.** 1980 Fall;14(3):383-408.

The relationship between geographic mobility, kinship ties and social status ˜is examined in this article using data from a sample of 820 **Mexican** immigrants aged 18 to 60, who were interviewed upon legal entry to the United States in late 1973-74, and reinterviewed three years later. An attempt is made to determine whether and how the maintenance of kinship ties influences the integration of immigrants during the period immediately following emigration. Some former studies show that maintaining close family ties facilitates the adjustment and eventual incorporation of migrants into the formal structures of the receiving community, while others indicate that intensive interaction with kin may slow the process of socioeconomic assimilation. A third group of studies shows that kinship is irrelevant to subsequent success. The findings of this study do not support the argument that the maintenance of ascriptive ties in the host environment hinders the socioeconomic assimilation of Mexican immigrants, but neither do they indicate that immigrants who can and do benefit from the assistance provided by kin in the host society are in an advantaged position vis-a-vis those who are not afforded such alternatives. The data do reinforce the importance of ascriptive ties for providing a support network that links immigrants with the host society prior to the actual move and during the early adjustment period. Results indicate that familism apparently has little to do with the process by which immigrants are assimilated into the formal structures of the U.S. economy, or more specifically, their status attainments in the host setting. Rather, the analysis suggests that the functions of family relationships may be more directly tied to the costs of the reproduction of the social relations in a capitalist economy than to the needs of the immigrants themselves.

122. *Tittle CK. Career, marriage, and family: values in adult roles and guidance. **Personnel and Guidance Journal.** 1982 Nov;61 (3):154-8.

This paper discusses the development of marriage and parenthood values and reports the responses of 600 urban eleventh graders (blacks, Hispanics, and whites), to three sets of values: career, marriage, and family. The subjects responded to each value set in the course of an individual, highly structured interview. Results show that the greatest number of group differences for each value set were by sex, followed by socioeconomic status and ethnic group. For occupational values, males gave higher ratings than females to high income, leadership, and leisure; females gave higher ratings to helping others, variety, and work in their field of interest. With regard to marriage values, females gave higher ratings to financial security, emotional support, and prestige. Males gave higher ratings to a normal life, their own home, and a feeling of leadership. In terms of parenthood values, males gave higher ratings to respect for others, a stable marriage, and a tie to the future as important to the decision to become a parent. Females gave higher ratings to variety, friendship, and a chance to express love.

123. Veatch RM ; Henry M. Introduction. In: Veatch RM, ed. **Population policy and ethics: the American experience.** A Project of the Research Group on Ethics and Population of the Institute of Society, Ethics and the Life Sciences. New York City, Irvington Publishers. 1977. p. 1-14. (Population and Demography Series).

Commissioned articles on American values and population policy by individual members of a research group are summarized. Topics covered are: 1) the American values of freedom, justice, general welfare, and security/survival as they have impinged on population policy; 2) historical analysis of American legal and moral/political traditions as they affect population control; 3) opinions on population policy held by blacks, women, members of the new left, Hispanics (**Mexicans**), Native Americans, religious groups, businessmen, labor union members, welfare recipients, ecologists, population geneticists, and physicians; and 4) legal and ethical implications of specific population policies including immigration reduction and abortion. It is noted that a set of criteria drawn up by the entire research group for the evaluation of policy alternatives is also included.

124. Vega WA ; Hough RL ; Romero A. Family life patterns of Mexican Americans. In: Powell GD, ed. **The psychosocial development of minority group children.** New York, Brunner-Mazel. 1983. p. 194-215.

This paper reviews and summarizes existing literature on the **Mexican** American family. Attention was given to the social class structure and role content of Mexican American families and the values that reinforce the system of mutual support. Support system components were described as multidimensional, multipurpose, and buttressed by an explicit set of culturally derived expectations which are mediated by various demographic factors, especially acculturation and social class. Though cultural behaviors which typify the interactional patterns within many Mexican American households were reviewed, it must be acknowledged that the variations to be found in familial adaptation preclude any closure on this topic. The paper concludes with the presentation of a comprehensive research model for understanding the Mexican American family. This model details the factors normally considered in the literature as stressors, but relates them within a temporal framework that specifically recognizes the importance of life changes and life events as integral etiologic factors and processes in family life with correspondent outcomes.

125. Warwick DP ; Williamson N. Population policy and Spanish surnamed Americans. In: Veatch RM, ed. **Population policy and ethics: the American experience.** A Project of the Research Group on Ethics and Population of The Institute of Society, Ethics and the Life Sciences. New York City, Irvington Publishers. 1977. p. 211-35. (Population and Demography Series).

Americans of Spanish speaking origins seem to have similar

values regarding the family, sex role definitions, and children. An interesting finding is the limited sphere of marital communication, particularly in the area of family planning and sexual behavior, because of: 1) traditional views of femininity; 2) male fear of loss of dominance; and 3) fear of the wife's infidelity. Children also fill roles: 1) male offspring prove a father's manliness; 2) motherhood is considered a woman's most important function; and 3) prolonged infertility can lead women to fear of abandonment. Hispanics use two arguments against population control: fear of genocide, and belief in increased power through larger numbers. Other opposition includes a lack of information, Roman Catholic opposition, and the economic contribution made by working children. While **Puerto Rican** women have accepted sterilization measures, few **Mexican** American women have expressed interest. Neither group encourages male sterilization. Further population problems result from illegal immigration. Finally, undercounting as a result of inadequate census procedures has led to a lack of attention for the needs and the culture of this important minority group.

126. Waterman C ; Johnson D. The Chicana: traditional values in transition. Paper presented at the Speech Communication Association, San Antonio, Texas. November 12, 1979. (ERIC Document No. 184771).

The Chicana has traditionally been seen as a silent partner in a marriage and culture: one who is totally subservient to her husband and devoted only to his needs and her children's needs. This research questions if this role is changing and, if so, how and to what degree. The Chicana has practically been paralyzed by the stereotyped identity awarded to her by the dominant reference group. The importance of this role as housewife and mother has been overlooked; her power in the domestic sphere is extensive and the **Mexican** American household can be defined as matrifocal. The Chicana is making adjustments in her role that coincide with the implementation of the sweeping social changes in the 1960s and 1970s in the United States: increased educational attainment is allowing upward socioeconomic mobility, weakened influence of the Catholic Church is changing attitudes about birth control and a woman's role outside the home, and increased intermarriage of Hispanics with non-Hispanics is resulting in cultural melding. However, there exists a common desire among those interviewed to maintain and preserve cultural identity. In part of that heritage resides a deep commitment to the home and family.

127. Weisbord RG. Strength in numbers: an old and oft-told tale. In: Weisbord RG. **Genocide? Birth control and the black American.** Westport, Connecticut, Greenwood Press. 1975. p. 56-75.

The ideology of strength in numbers is not exclusively found in black Americans. Various national, racial, religious, and ethnic groups have historically been concerned with the long term effects of birth control. Such groups as **Mexican** Americans, Nazis, post World War II French, American Indians, and **South Americans** are cited as examples of groups opposing birth control on the grounds of reduced group strength. On the zero population growth issue, Joe C. Ortega, a staff counsel for the Mexican American Legal Defense and Educational Fund, has found his people simultaneously pulled in opposite directions. Fewer Chicanos would mean more jobs and a fairer share of America's

wealth.   On the other hand, zero population growth could under-
mine the deeply rooted traditions of a close, large family.   If
Puerto Rico were to have a natural growth rate of two percent,
by the year 2000 its density would be comparable to squeezing
double the world's present population into the United States.
Puerto Rican groups favoring independence for their crowded
Caribbean island rather than the existing commonwealth status
insist that an independent, sovereign Puerto Rican state would
benefit from and could support a still larger population.

128. Williams JE. Some findings about the impact of sex roles
on definitions of rape for Anglos, blacks and Mexican Americans.
Paper of the Society for the Study of Social Problems. (Unpublished) 1978.

The relationship between sex role attitudes and attitudes about
rape is examined for three different racial/ethnic groups:
Anglos, blacks and **Mexican** Americans. It was hypothesized that
attitudes about traditional sex roles and women's liberation
could account for attitudes about rape over and above what may
be accounted for by such socioeconomic variables as age, sex,
education, and income. Based on sex role differences, historical experience with rape, the criminal justice system, and
differential exposure to the consciousness raising of the women's movement, ethnic/racial groups were expected to differ in
their attitudes about rape. The purpose here was thus: to
examine sex role attitudes vis-a-vis rape; and to develop models
which best predict (for each ethnic group) feminist/liberal
attitudes about rape. Based on a combination of the best socioeconomic status predictors and sex role/women's liberation predictors of attitudes about rape, some tentative models are
developed, predictive of liberal/feminist attitudes about rape
for each of the three racial/ethnic groups. Comparisons are
drawn among the groups, and some explanation is offered for the
differences.

129. Williams JE ; Holmes KA. **Rape: the public view** – **the**
personal experience. Final Report. National Institute for Mental
Health Grant. 1979. 540 p.

An exploration of the interplay between society and the personal
experience of rape is presented based on a theory of racial/
sexual stratification which leads to a view of rape as the convergence of racism and sexism. Part I is based on data from
over 1,000 personal interviews representing three racial/ethnic
(Anglo, black, and **Mexican** American) communities in the City of
San Antonio, Texas. An empirical description of public attitudes about rape, specified by race/ethnicity and sex, and an
investigation of the empirical associations between attitudes
about rape and sex role/race related attitudes is presented.
Part II describes a sample of rape victims in order to assess
the impact of their experience, and to examine their perceptions
of needs, services and support systems. It is suggested that
there are significant differences in the impact of the rape
experience related to race/ethnicity impacts which take on
social clarity principally against the reality of community
attitudes.

130. Wood CH ; Bean FD. Offspring gender and family size:
implications from a comparison of Mexican Americans and Anglo
Americans. **Journal of Marriage and the Family.** 1977 Feb;39(1):
129-39.

The questions of whether and how offspring gender preferences affect eventual family size assume greater proportions given recent technological developments in reproductive gender control and given the trend in the United States toward preferences for smaller families. Using 1970 U.S. Census Public Use Sample data for Anglos and **Mexican** Americans, this study examines the relationship between the gender of children already born and the likelihood of having subsequent children. The results indicate that couples with previous children of the same gender are consistently more likely to bear an additional child compared to those with a gender mix. Though present among members of both groups, this relationship is more pronounced among Anglos than Mexican Americans. The effects of the wife's education on the likelihood of another birth are also examined and found to be greater among couples with a gender mix than among those with children of the same gender. The relevance of these findings to the issue of what kinds of wives opt to have fewer children is discussed. The trend toward families of smaller sizes may heighten parental interest in the gender of early born children.

3. Marriage and Household Structure

The prevalence of extended families and a special appreciation of close family ties is one popular stereotype of Hispanic families which tends to be borne out by research. In part because of migration, Hispanic families also tend to have high rates of **female-headed households.** In these households, particularly where there are children, **extended familism** may be a means of coping and making up for support from the absent spouse.

Other topics examined in this section include studies of **intermarriage** of Hispanics and Anglos, and of persons of different Hispanic origins, and of the use of intermarriage as a measure of acculturation. While rates of intermarriage between Mexican origin and Anglo Americans are increasing, the continued influx of new Mexican immigrants presents a deterrent to the absorption of this population into the majority society.

Other researchers have examined what appears to be the lower likelihood of Hispanics, particularly Mexican origin couples, to face **marital instability.**

131. Aguirre BE. The marital stability of Cubans in the United States. **Ethnicity.** 1981 Dec;8(4):387-405.

The importance of the Cuban Revolution of 1959 for understanding **Cuban** immigrant marriages in the United States is underscored with an empirical typology of marriages of Cuban immigrants devised from country, year of first marriage, and year of immigration. The typology is used in the Multiple Classification Analysis of the marital stability of Cuban men and women in the Five Percent Public Use National Sample of the 1970 U.S. Census. A set of theoretically specified predictors of marital instability is used. The results indicate inapplicability of the institutional marriage ideal type in explaining the correlates of marital instability among Cuban immigrants. Needed research is suggested. Male refugees first married in Cuba, and females first married in the U.S. after the revolution, have very stable

marriages.   Nearness of residence to the culture of origin, to
kin, and extent of assimilation are insignificant predictors of
marital instability in most marriage cohorts.   Conflicting results occur when the effects on marital instability of the
instrumental abilities of males and females (as measured by
their health, education, occupation, and income), and the fertility of the latter, are analyzed.   The relative modernity of
the marriages of Cubans in the U.S. is noted.

132.   Arce CH ; Abney GA. Demographic and cultural correlates of
Chicano intermarriage. **California Sociologist.** 1982 Summer;5(2):
41-57.

Previous studies of Chicano intermarriage have concentrated on
structural variables.   A sociopsychological investigation of
intermarriage is presented, with emphasis on language maintenance, religious preference, choice of ethnic label, and childrearing customs.   Data were obtained from an interview survey of
Mexican Americans (720 currently married, 127 formerly married;
330 male, 497 female) from Arizona, California, New Mexico,
Texas and metropolitan Chicago, Illinois conducted by Carlos H.
Arce and Robert Santos ("Design and Execution Problems in a Rare
Population Sample Survey," unpublished paper, Survey Research
Center, University of Michigan).   The results show that the
exogamous Chicanos are on the average two years younger than the
endogamous.   Moreover, those who intermarry have three more
years of education and a higher income than those who do not.
About 75% of the exogamous Chicanos are United States natives,
compared to 60% of the endogamous.   Religion had little effect
on intermarriage.   Endogamous Chicanos were more likely to claim
Spanish as their main language.

133.   Cazares RB ; Murguia E ; Frisbie WP.   Mexican American
intermarriage in a nonmetropolitan context. **Social Science Quarterly.** 1984 Jun;65(2):626-34.

Intermarriage has long been viewed as a measure of a group's
social distance and as an indicator of the maintenance of ethnic
boundaries.   Rates of exogamy indicate the amount of a given
group's assimilation into a larger and dominant group's social
structure.   Examination of marriage records in Pecos County,
Texas, from 1880 to 1978 shows an overall outmarriage rate of
.091 for marriages and .048 for individuals, documenting the
considerable social distance that historically has existed between **Mexican** and Anglo American residents of this region.
However, intermarriage rates rose significantly after 1970.
This recent increase in exogamy suggests a notable lessening of
normative proscriptions concerning majority/minority contact in
at least one area of the non-metropolitan southwest.   To the
extent that this county is representative of other non-
metropolitan areas throughout the southwest, this finding could
signal the beginning of real change in Anglo/Chicano relationships in non-urban areas, regions where minority/majority social
distance has historically been very great.

134.   *Cherlin A ; McCarthy J. Remarried couple households. Presented at the 52nd Annual Meeting of the Population Association
of America, Pittsburgh, Pennsylvania. April 14-16, 1983. (Unpublished) 21 p.

The June 1980 Current Population Survey (CPS), collected information on 173,229 people in 62,992 households.   Using the public

release tape from the June 1980 CPS, all households were identified in which a currently married husband and wife were enumerated, and in which both the husband and wife were between the
ages of 15 and 75, and either the husband or the wife or both
had been divorced prior to the start of the current marriage.
Race, Hispanic ethnicity, years of school completed, and age
were the only four permanent background characteristics about
which information was collected.   In one-fifth of all households
in the United States in June 1980 maintained by a married couple, both aged 15 to 75, one or both spouses had been divorced.
One-fifth of all children under 18 living in married couple
households, and about one-sixth of all children under 18 in the
U.S., were in households in which one or both spouses had remarried following a divorce.   In about two-thirds of the remarried
couples in which the husband was under 40, at least one spouse
had children under 18 from a previous marriage, but few reported
having all three possible sets of children under 18 (from both
previous marriages and from the current marriage).

135. Cooney RS. Demographic components of growth in white,
black, and Puerto Rican female-headed families: comparison of
the Cutright and Ross/Sawhill methodologies. **Social Science
Research.** 1979;8(2):144-58.

In 1970, 96% of maritally disrupted **Puerto Rican** women with
children under age 18 were heads of households.   The percentage
for never married women with children was 90.   The direction of
the change in these figures between 1960 and 1970 is the same
for Puerto Ricans and non-Hispanic blacks and whites.   That is,
ever married heads of households have increased and never married heads have decreased.   This study examines the methodological differences between Cutright's and Ross/Sawhill's analyses
of the demographic components of change in these numbers and
replicates their procedures within a comparable time/age framework in order to resolve their contradictory findings.   The
analysis suggests that while changes in marital instability and
living arrangements are the two major factors accounting for
changes in the number of white female-headed families between
1960 and 1970, the two most important demographic components for
Puerto Ricans and blacks related to these are population growth
and the increased likelihood that children were present in the
home when marital disruption occurred.

136.   *Cooney RS ;   Min K. Demographic characteristics affecting
living arrangements among young currently unmarried Puerto
Rican, non-Spanish black, and non-Spanish white mothers. **Ethnicity.** 1981 Jun;8(2):197-200.

Two research questions were addressed in this study: 1) what
sociodemographic variables affect the living arrangements of
young currently unmarried mothers, aged 14 to 29, within ethnic/
racial groups; and 2) how successfully do these variables
account for the large ethnic/racial differences in headship
probabilities among **Puerto Ricans,** whites, and blacks.   Three
factors: number of children, migration status and education
derived from Sweet's (1972) earlier work were used in concep-
tualizing the relevance of sociodemographic characteristics to
headship probabilities among young and currently unmarried
mothers.   The data were drawn from the 1-in-100 Public Use
Sample tapes for the New York metropolitan region in 1970.
Study focus was on young, aged 14 to 29, maritally disrupted, or
never married mothers in the New York metropolitan area in 1970.

Puerto Ricans showed a higher probability than both blacks and whites to head their own households, and blacks showed a higher probability than whites.   Study findings demonstrated that migration status affects the headship probabilities of young currently unmarried Puerto Rican, black and white mothers.   Number of children and migration status accounted for the major differences in headship probabilities between whites and blacks, and migration status and education accounted for the major differences between Puerto Ricans and blacks.

137. Eberstein IW ; Frisbie WP. Differences in marital instability among Mexican Americans, blacks, and Anglos: 1960 and 1970. **Social Problems.** 1976 Jun;23(5):609-21.

The purpose of this research is twofold: to investigate changes in **Mexican** American marital solidarity with respect to blacks and Anglos that may have occurred between 1960 and 1970, and to examine predictions made by Uhlenberg premised on the analysis of 1960 data.   Uhlenberg's 1972 research is developed and then assessed on the basis of data for both 1960 and 1970.   The data were obtained primarily from the 1960 and 1970 1-in-100 Public Use Samples for five southwestern states and supplemented by published census materials.   The entire Mexican American and black ever married female populations, aged 20 to 64, included in the Public Use Samples for these five states were studied as well as a ten percent subsample of Anglo ever married females, aged 20 to 64, for the same region.   It appears that Mexican American women are least likely and black women are most likely to have a history of marital dissolution. This ranking persists with controls for age, age at first marriage, education, and place of residence.   The proportionate increase in marital instability recorded by Anglo women between 1960 and 1970 is larger than that for either Mexican American or black women.

138. Farrell J ; Markides KS. Marriage and health: A threegeneration study of Mexican Americans. **Journal of Marriage and the Family.** 1985 Nov:1029-36.

The relationships between health and marital status and marital satisfaction were investigated with data from a three-generation study of **Mexican** Americans. Overall, few consistent differences in physical health symptoms and self-rated health were found by marital status once effects of sex, age, income, and education were held constant.   The few significant differences found were generally in the middle and younger generations.   Women were found to report poorer health than men in all generations. When married people were examined separately, it was found that marital satisfaction was not related to the health of the older generation, but was in the middle and younger generation (controlling for other variables).   The associations were stronger for the younger generation.   It was concluded that marriage and good marriage appear to have more protective influences on younger Mexican Americans, though the possibility was acknowledged that generational differences may reflect selection effects.

139. Frisbie WP ; Bean FD ; Eberstein IW. Patterns of marital instability among Mexican Americans, blacks, and Anglos. In: Bean FD and Frisbie WP, eds. **Studies in population: The demography of racial and ethnic groups.** New York City, Academic Press. 1978. p. 143-64.

The data utilized in this research were obtained from the 1970 1-in-100 (five percent) Public Use Samples for five southwestern states: Arizona,   California,   Colorado,   New Mexico,   and Texas. The research focused upon three hypotheses implicit in the literature dealing with racial/ethnic group differences in marital instability for **Mexican** Americans,   blacks and Anglos.   The analysis suggests that neither ethnicity specific nor socioeconomic factors alone are adequate explanations of these differentials,   but   that   these two sets of variables interact   in   the determination of racial/ethnic differences in family solidarity. However,   only partial support is evident for this conclusion,   in that   the relationship between age at first marriage and marital instability varies significantly by race/ethnicity,   although the relationship between education and marital instability does not. Additional   investigation is necessary to ascertain more clearly the   relative   validity of these three perspectives   on   racial/ ethnic differences in family dissolution.

140. *Frisbie WP ;   Bean FD ;   Eberstein IW.   Recent changes in marital   instability among Mexican Americans: convergence   with black and Anglo trends? **Social Forces.** 1980 Jun;58(4):1205-20.

Cohort analysis is applied to Public Use Samples for five southwestern   states   from the 1960 and 1970 United States Censuses, yielding   samples of 82,827 and 102,055 Anglo;   7,013 and 9,610 black;   and 10,149 and 13,818 **Mexican** American women aged 15 and over   to   determine   comparative changes in   the   prevalence   of marital   instability among the three groups.   Analyses of   detailed   categories of marital status,   and a summary measure   of instability,   reveal   that   women in all three   groups   recorded increases in marital dissolution.   However,   differences in increase rates,   especially among the younger cohorts,   suggest a difference in trend,   indicating an overall divergence.   Lessened differentials   were more common between blacks and   Anglos   than between blacks and Mexican Americans.   One possible interpretation of the persistence of the differentials over time has to do with the distinctive cultural milieu which some attribute to the Mexican American population.

141. Frisbie WP ;   Bean FD ;   Kaufman R ;   Mutchler J. Nativity and   household/family structure among the Mexican origin population of the United States.   Austin,   Texas,   University of Texas, Texas Population Research Center.   1984.   25 plus unnumbered   p. (Texas Population Research Center Paper No. 6.008).

This   paper is concerned with the household and family structure of immigrants from Mexico in the United States.   In particular, comparisons are made between the household and family structural patterns   of legal **Mexican** immigrants and those of   native   born persons   of Mexican origin.   Changes between 1960 and 1970   are also considered.   The data are from the 1960 and 1970 Public Use Sample   Micro Data files of the U.S.   Census.   While there were substantial   differences   between native born and   foreign   born Mexican Americans as recently as 1960,   a remarkable convergence in household structure patterns occurred in the ensuing   decades such that,   by 1980,   there were few major differences separating either   the two immigrant status populations from each other or, for that matter,   from Anglos.   One type of change   responsible for   the bulk of the striking convergence of trends,   is seen in the shifting patterns of co-residence among the native born, who followed the general trend in the U.S.   toward higher levels   of marital instability,   greater prevalence of female-headed households, and fewer households with large numbers of children. Lastly, the structure and composition of illegal immigrant households are not such as to suggest a weak or unstable organization.

142. *Frisbie WP ; Bean FD ; Poston DL ; Kaufman R. Changes in Hispanic household/family structure. Austin, Texas, University of Texas, Texas Population Research Center. 1983. 31 p. (Texas Population Research Center Paper No. 5.005).

This paper reports on an application of standardization techniques for contingency tables to adjust for life cycle composition as it affects household/family patterns among household/family types that distinguish **Mexican** Americans, **Puerto Ricans,** and **Cubans** from each other and from non-Hispanic whites and blacks.   Data from the 1960 and 1970 Public Use Samples are used.   Some results are: 1) while life cycle effects are substantial, strong racial/ethnic differences in household structure remain after adjusting for life cycle stage; 2) persons are more likely to live alone at young ages; 3) a household containing an only and widowed female is more likely for women aged 65 and over than of other ages; 4) never disrupted households with no children are more concentrated in the younger ages; 5) never disrupted households are more typical of Hispanic than of Anglo or black groups; 6) Cubans have the greatest likelihood of being in a never disrupted household; 7) Mexican Americans are not likely to be in one person female-headed or widow-headed households; and 8) there is a high likelihood of never married females with children among Puerto Ricans.

143. Frisbie WP ; Inman JM ; Poston DL ; Bean FD. Household and family demography of Hispanics: a comparative analysis. Austin, Texas, University of Texas, Texas Population Research Center. 1982. 33 plus unnumbered p. (Texas Population Research Center Paper No. 4.002).

Patterns of household composition and family structure among **Mexican, Puerto Rican, Cuban,** black, and Anglo populations in the United States are analyzed using variables such as sex, age of family members, family size, kinship, and marital status. Also investigated are the changes in household/family structure that took place between 1960 and 1970.   Data are from the 1-in-100 Public Use Samples of the 1960 and 1970 Censuses.   Some government documents and certain pieces of research have treated all Hispanics (i.e., those of Spanish origin) as a single, undifferentiated ethnic entity, presumably on the grounds that their Latin American origin has provided them with a common language, religion, and a similar cultural heritage.   But a closer inspection of the subgroups that make up the Hispanic population casts doubt on the suitability of this approach. When the Hispanic population is disaggregated, approximately 60% is of Mexican background, 14% is Puerto Rican, seven percent is Cuban, seven percent is Central or South American, and 11% is of other Spanish origin.

144. Frisbie WP ; McCall PL ; Mutchler J. The lonely crowd? An investigation of Hispanic participation in the rise of one person households. Austin, Texas, University of Texas, Texas Population Research Center. 1983. 24 p. (Texas Population Research Center Paper No. 5.006).

The purpose of this analysis is to explore in detail the extent to which **Mexicans, Puerto Ricans** and **Cubans** have participated in the emergence of one person households in the United States. Data from the 1960 and 1970 Public Use Sample Micro Data files were used. The authors found that for most, but not all Hispanic groups, the proportion of one person households increased between 1960 and 1970, but the increase was never more than two percent for any group. In contrast, the comparable percentages for Anglos and blacks rose by about 5%. Among Cubans there was actually a decline in the proportion. Except for Cubans, all groups experienced a decline in average size of household to go along with the increasing prevalence of persons living alone, but the composition of the decline varied greatly between Hispanic groups. A major difference distinguishing Hispanic groups is that the relative number of female-headed households in these groups is consistently below the percentage that is male-headed, while exactly the opposite is true of blacks and Anglos. The economic implications of living alone are discussed.

145. Frisbie WP ; Mutchler J ; Poston DL ; Kelly WR ; Browning HL ; Krivo LJ ; Bean FD. Household family structure and socio-economic differentials: a comparison of Hispanics, blacks and Anglos. Austin, Texas, University of Texas, Texas Population Research Center. 1982. 27 p. (Texas Population Research Center Paper No. 4.009).

The purpose of this analysis is to compare the status of the three major Hispanic populations in the United States (**Mexicans, Puerto Ricans** and **Cubans**) along several significant socioeconomic and sociodemographic dimensions: comparisons are also made with Anglo and non-Hispanic black populations. The data for the analysis were drawn from the 1960 1-in-100 Public Use Sample and from a 3-in-100 Sample compiled from the 1970 Public Use Sample five percent questionnaire. Findings are presented for the following characteristics: distribution of household/family types, household size by race/ethnicity, education, labor force participation and employment status, occupation and income, and home ownership. The authors conclude that not only are there substantial differences in household/family structure across the Hispanic groups, but also that these differences are likely to remain for some time along with concommitant variations in the socioeconomic characteristics of these populations.

146. *Frisbie WP ; Opitz W. Race/ethnic and gender differentials in marital instability: 1980. Austin, Texas, University of Texas, Population Research Center. 1985. 18 p. (Texas Population Research Center Paper No. 7.007).

This research examines the prevalence of marital disruption among **Mexican** Americans, blacks, and non-Hispanic whites in 1980 while taking into account gender differentials associated with differences in mortality and immigration. Through log-linear analysis of data drawn from the 1980 Public Use Micro Data ·(File A), it was demonstrated that Mexican Americans of both sexes have substantially higher odds of intact marriages, while blacks of both sexes have the lowest odds of marital stability. Young age at marriage acts to substantially decrease the chances of a stable marital union. The finding of a greater prevalence of marital dissolution at intermediate levels of education holds for Anglos and blacks, but not for Mexican Americans. The effect is also absent in the low age at marriage category where there is a monotonic decline in stability odds as education increases. A plausible interpretation of the former interaction is that education acts to reduce the ties of Mexican Americans to traditional familistic values.   The latter interaction may result from increased levels of stress occasioned by the pursuit of advanced education among persons who marry as teenagers.

147. Frisbie WP ; Opitz W ; Kelly WR. Marital instability trends among Mexican Americans as compared to blacks and Anglos: new evidence. **Social Science Quarterly.** 1985 Sep;66(3):587-601.

This research investigates both the current levels of marital instability among **Mexican** American, black, and Anglo women in the southwest, and trends in marital disruption between 1960 and 1980.   The data clearly indicate that the overall trend was one of increasing marital dissolution in the 1960-80 interval. Mexican American women consistently have the lowest prevalence of marital instability, and there is no convergence of the Mexican American pattern with either the black or Anglo trends. Significant racial/ethnic differentials persist net of the effects of current age, age at marriage and socioeconomic status.

148. Gurak DT ; Fitzpatrick JP. Intermarriage among Hispanic ethnic groups in New York City. **American Journal of Sociology.** 1982 Jan;87(4):921-34.

Intermarriage provides an excellent indicator of assimilation and of the social distance separating ethnic groups. Using 1975 marriage records this report describes the intermarriage patterns of five Hispanic groups in New York City.   Of the 27,712 Hispanics included in these marriages, 56% were **Puerto Rican,** 19% were **South Americans,** 13% were **Dominicans,** 8% were **Mexicans** or **Central Americans,** and 4% were **Cubans.**   The tendency for Hispanics to marry within their own national origin group varies considerably among the five Hispanic groups.   Particularly for the second generation, there are high rates of outgroup marriage, both with other Hispanics and with non-Hispanics. Puerto Ricans provide a major exception to this pattern, having low rates of outgroup marriage in both generations.   A control for group size does not explain the low Puerto Rican second generation rate.   A comparison with 1949 and 1959 data indicates that an earlier trend toward Puerto Rican marital assimilation has reversed.   Several possible explanations for the Puerto Rican pattern are suggested.

149. Gurak DT ; Kritz MM. Dominican and Colombian women in New York City: household structure and employment patterns. **Migration Today.** 1982;10(3-4):14-21.

This article provides a profile of the household structure and labor force participation of **Dominican** and **Colombian** women in New York City using data from a 1981 probability survey.   The survey included interviews with a probability sample of 900 Colombian and Dominican men and women and obtained information on legal status at entry, migration histories, family structure, and employment experience.   Recent data from a sample survey of Colombian and Dominican immigrants in New York City show significant differences between immigrant women in their background characteristics, household structure, and employment patterns. Compared to their Dominican counterparts, Colombian women tend to migrate at an older age, be more urban in background, and have more employment experience prior to migration. Experiences in the United States also differ.   Colombian women are more likely to be a part of a nuclear family household and to be employed in 1981. In contrast, Dominican women have a much higher proportion of single parent households and receiving public assistance. The preponderance of women among U.S. immigrants and the distinctive patterns identified among these two Hispanic groups indicates the importance of addressing further research into the characteristics of female immigrants, and their settlement and acculturation processes.

150. Kearl MC ; Murguia E. Age differences of spouses in Mexican American intermarriage: exploring the cost of minority assimilation. **Social Science Quarterly.** 1985 Jun;66(2):453-60.

One widely recognized indicator of minority assimilation into the majority society is intermarriage between minority and majority groups. Using marriage certificates from three areas in the southwest, this study considers the costs of minority members entering into exogamous unions with a spouse from the majority culture. Age differences are used as a measure of spouse power inequalities to test the hypothesis that **Mexican** Americans entering into exogamous marriages yield the age advantages they would have had in endogamous unions. In general, this hypothesis is confirmed for females, but not for males. Contrary to expectations, Spanish surnamed males were found typically to have greater age advantages within exogamous relationships although, as predicted, both Hispanic and Anglo women generally had greater age similarity with them than with Anglo spouses. In general, increasing age at marriage for males greatly increases their age advantage over their spouses, but the results are not as clear for females. A previous divorce tends to diminish male age advantage except in the case of endogamous non-Spanish surnamed couples.

151. Keefe SE. Real and ideal extended familism among Mexican Americans and Anglo Americans: on the meaning of close family ties. **Human Organization.** 1984 Spring;43(1):65-70.

Research conducted in three southern California cities suggests that **Mexican** Americans tend to have traditional extended families marked by geographic proximity, while Anglos tend to have modified extended families with little geographic proximity. Despite differences in extended family structure, however, both ethnic groups score relatively high on an extended family value scale. It is suggested that the critical difference between the two ethnic groups is in the meaning of close family ties. Mexican Americans require the consistent presence of family members while Anglos are content with intermittent visits supplemented by telephone calls and letters. Thus, Anglos can value familism that is defined so as to permit considerable geographic mobility. It is argued that this difference in familial values and preference for geographic stability are not necessarily linked with socioeconomic factors. There is no evidence that Mexican Americans' lower socioeconomic status is the product of differences in extended familism as either a value or behavioral system.

152. Markides KS ; Hoppe SK. Marital satisfaction in three generations of Mexican Americans. **Social Science Quarterly.** 1985 Mar;66(1):147-54.

This paper replicates Gilford and Bengtson's analysis of marital satisfaction in three generations with data from a three-generation study of **Mexican** Americans. As in the earlier study, members of the younger generation have the highest marital satisfaction. However, unlike the Gilford and Bengtson findings, there is a U-shaped satisfaction curve across the life cycle only for men. For women, successively lower marital satisfaction levels from younger to older generations are observed. On three other single item indicators, high levels of marital satisfaction are observed in the older generation, with women being somewhat less satisfied.

153.   *Mindel CH. Extended familism among urban Mexican Americans, Anglos, and blacks. **Hispanic Journal of Behavioral Science**. 1980;2(1):21-34.

The data for this study were collected in 1974 as part of a larger investigation of a tri-ethnic and geographically isolated urban community in Kansas City, Missouri. The research design called for a purposive sample of parents with at least one child enrolled in a neighbornood elementary school. Complete data were obtained for 143 Anglos, 160 blacks and 152 **Mexican** Americans. The measure of extended familism used in this study has four indices: extensity of presence, intensity of presence, interaction and functionality. The data clearly indicate that the Anglos in this sample maintain the lowest level of extended familism on all four measures. Mexican Americans appear to have larger families, and therefore, engage in more extensive kinship. Blacks, on the other hand, appear to have smaller families and interact with them less, but use their kin in a more instrumental fashion as a mutual aid and support system. The pattern that emerges concerning migration is that Anglos migrate away from their kin network whereas blacks and, to an even greater extent, Mexican Americans migrate within a kin network. For blacks and Mexican Americans, the functional and/or cultural requirements lead to a much more kinship involved family pattern.

154.   Mittelbach FG ; Moore JW. Ethnic endogamy: the case of Mexican Americans. **American Journal of Sociology**. 1968;74(1):50-62.

A three-generational analysis of marriages involving **Mexican** Americans shows higher rates of exogamy than do earlier studies. The analysis is based on approximately 7,500 marriage licenses issued in Los Angeles County during 1963 in which one or both spouses had a Spanish surname. Exogamy is higher for women and increases with removal from immigrant status. There is a strong pattern of generational endogamy and a strong suggestion that social distance between generations may be as important as social distance between the ethnic group and the dominant society. Exogamy is more prevalent among higher status individuals. With some exceptions, occupation appears to be a better predictor of exogamy than generation. Generally, the older the groom, the more "Mexican" the spouse, though the pattern is not the same for brides. Findings have implications for assimilation of Mexican Americans and for understanding processes of assimilation.

155.   Murguia E ; Cazares RB. Intermarriage of Mexican Americans. In: **Intermarriage in the United States**. Hawthorne Press. 1982. p. 91-100.

This study presents empirical evidence on the changing intermarriage rates for **Mexican** Americans. In the long run the authors feel it is difficult to imagine anything but an overall slow increase in rates of Chicano intermarriage, as Chicanos in increasing numbers reach middle class status. As this population moves out of ethnic enclaves (barrios), it moves in the direction of increasing contact on an equal basis with the majority population. On the other hand, there are three factors which for the foreseeable future will keep the Chicano population from complete absorption into the majority society. First is that the group is, in part, non-Caucasian and therefore physically distinct from and identifiable by the majority. Racial differences are among the strongest barriers to the development of primary relationships and subsequent intermarriage between groups. Second, there is the continuing immigration of both documented and undocumented workers from Mexico to the United States. First generation Chicanos have a lower rate of outmarriage than do subsequent generations. Finally, the close proximity to Mexico provides continuing contact and continuous movement back and forth across the border; this has the effect of limiting absorption through intermarriage.

156. Murguia E ; Frisbie WP. Trends in Mexican American intermarriage: recent findings in perspective. **Social Science Quarterly.** 1977;59(3):374-89.

This research focuses on the intermarriage patterns of the Spanish surnamed (**Mexican** American) population with the non-Spanish surnamed population, over time, for a number of different locations (mainly urban centers) throughout the southwestern United States. A 20% random sample of marriage applications recorded in Bernadillo County was drawn for each of the years 1967 and 1971 (n=1385). A ten percent random sample of marriage applications recorded in Bear County was drawn for each of the years 1964, 1967, 1971, and 1973 (n=3505). Observed intermarriage rates are studied in conjunction with expected rates calculated as probabilities based on the size of the minority relative to the total population marrying. Without doubt, Spanish surnamed exogamy rates have increased over time in the southwest, but the trend has been slow to develop. If the level of Spanish surnamed intermarriage is conceived as the most conclusive, objective indicator of the degree of assimilation of the minority, it seems probable that the Mexican American population will continue to represent a distinct sociocultural entity for some time to come.

157. Rogler LH ; Cooney RS. **Puerto Rican families in New York City: intergenerational processes.** Maplewood, New Jersey, Waterfront Press. 1985. 211 p.

The integration of immigrant groups into American society has been widely researched, but little is known about the relationship between a migration induced change in the sociocultural environment of parents and their children, and intergenerational processes within the family. This book examines the lives of 100 intergenerationally linked **Puerto Rican** families in New York City. Each family consists of the married parents and their married child and spouse. Intergenerational differences in ethnic identity, spouse relationships, and socioeconomic mobility are explored.

158. Schoen R ; Nelson VE ; Collins M. Intermarriage among Spanish surnamed Californians: 1962-1974. **International Migration Review.** 1978;12(3):359-69.

The nature and extent of outgroup marriage among **Mexican** Americans in California during the 1962-74 period is analyzed here
through marriage records coded to indicate the Spanish surname
status of the bride and groom.   A high level of outmarriage was
found, on the order of one-third to two-fifths of those marrying.   Differentials in outmarriage proportions by age and sex
were examined and tended to be relatively small.   More substantial differentials were found with regard to marriage order,
where higher order marriages of Spanish surnamed persons were
more likely than first marriages to involve a non-Spanish surnamed partner.   The largest differentials were generational,
with Spanish surnamed persons not born in Mexico much more
likely to outmarry than were those born in Mexico.   The dominant
impression that emerges from the data is that the major trends
and differentials in the Spanish surnamed group are closely
linked to immigration from Mexico.

159.   *Sweet JA.   Changes in marital status and living arrangements of adults: blacks and Mexican Americans. Madison, Wisconsin, University of Wisconsin. 1979. 21 p. (Center for Demography
and Ecology Working Paper No. 79-16).

This paper examines the household living arrangements of young
unmarried black and Chicano (**Mexican**) adults aged 18 to 24.
Data are compared for the years 1960 and 1970. Rising levels of
education and increased levels of school enrollment made it
essential to disaggregate the populations by education.   The
following is a summary of the changes found among the total
Hispanic sample between 1960 and 1970.   The proportion of never
married males who did not complete high school decreased, the
proportion of those who were high school graduates increased,
and there was no change for those enrolled in college.   The
corresponding statistics for females were increases for both
less than high school graduates and high school graduates, and
no change for those enrolled in college.   There was a small
increase in the percent single for males aged 18 to 19 and a
small decrease for those aged 20 to 24.   The percent single
increased for females of all ages.   The major changes in living
arrangements were an increase in the proportion of men in the
parental household, but a slight decrease for women, and a
decrease in the proportion of men in other group quarters, but a
slight increase for women.

160.   Tienda M ; Angel R. Headship and household composition
among blacks, Hispanics, and other whites. **Social Forces**. 1982
Dec;6(12):508-31.

A 1976 survey of income and education data was used to examine
differences in the prevalence of extended household structure
(EHS) among black, Hispanic (**Mexican, Puerto Rican, Central
American, South American**), and non-Hispanic white female-headed
and husband/wife households.   Results indicate that the greater
prevalence of EHS among Hispanics and blacks was related to
cultural circumstances and the attempt of households to cope
with economic hardship.   Female headship, frequently associated
with economic disadvantage, was significantly related to a higher incidence of EHS, which may also indicate a greater incentive
to find surrogate replacements for absent spouses.   Findings
suggest that the cultural variant explanation of EHS deserves
closer scrutiny in the analysis of family organization among
racial and ethnic groups.

161. Uhlenberg P. Marital instability among Mexican Americans:
following the patterns of blacks. **Social Problems.** 1972 Summer;
20(1):49-56.

While existing literature repeatedly states that rates of marital instability are low among **Mexican** Americans, data from the
1960 United States Census are analyzed to show that this is not
so.   A comparison of subgroups defined by generation and place
of residence is presented. The evidence suggests that instability among third generation Mexican Americans living in California is producing a pattern similar to that now characteristic of
blacks. As among blacks, the inability of many Mexican American
males to adequately provide for their families at the level they
deem necessary, due to low wages and widespread unemployment,
appears to be an important source of marital strain.   While
increasing marital instability may be viewed as an adaptation to
their current deprived circumstances, it is also possible that
it may hinder the group's future economic advancement.   An
increase in the number of broken homes will retard the achievement of future generations. The 1970 census data will allow for
a more adequate assessment of the trend in marital instability
within the large Mexican American population.

162. *U.S. Department of Commerce, Bureau of the Census. Families maintained by female householders: 1970-1979. By: Rawlings
SW. **Current Population Reports.** 1980;P-23(iv). 53 p.

This report provides United States data on female householders
with rro husband present and their families during the decade of
the 1970s.   Data are included on characteristics such as age,
race, Spanish origin, number and age of children, place of
residence, marital status, education, employment status, occupation, mobility, and income. Among whites, 12% of all families
were maintained by female householders in 1979. By contrast 41%
of black families and 20% of Spanish origin families were maintained by women.   Black and Spanish origin women maintaining
families were more likely than were women maintaining families
in the general population to be concentrated in and around
cities;   80% of black and 90% of Spanish origin women lived in
metropolitan areas.   Between 1970 and 1979, the median age of
white female householders declined by 6.8 years from 50.5 to
43.7 years; however, they were still likely to be somewhat older
than their black or Spanish origin counterparts. Families maintained by black women in 1979 were larger on the average   (3.63
persons) than those maintained by either Spanish origin women
(3.30 persons) or white women (2.86 persons).

163. *U.S. Department of Commerce, Bureau of the Census. Marital status and living arrangements: March 1981. **Current Population Reports** (CPR), Population Characteristics. 1982;P-20(372):
1-64; and ---, Marital status and living arrangements: March
1982. CPR, Population Characteristics. 1983 May;P-20(380); and
---, Marital status and living arrangements: March 1983. CPR,
Population Characteristics. 1984;P-20(389); and ---, Marital
status and living arrangements: March 1984. CPR, Population
Characteristics. 1985 Jul;P-20(399).

These reports present detailed statistics on the marital status
and living arrangements of persons in the non-institutional
population of the United States, based on the March Current
Population Survey. Generally, these statistics are presented by
age, sex, race, and Spanish origin. The text discusses changes

in the median age at first marriage, the proportion of young
adults never married, the divorce ratio, presence of parents for
persons under 18 years old, and persons living alone or with
unrelated persons.

164. Valdez A. Recent increases in intermarriage by Mexican
American males: Bexar County, Texas from 1971 to 1980. **Social
Science Quarterly.** 1983 Mar;64(1):136-44.

United States Census data and other official statistics for
Bexar County, Texas show that consistent with previous decades,
Mexican American exogamy rates during the 1970s steadily increased. However, this increase was a result of a rise in
outmarriage rates for Mexican American males rather than females, as was the case in the past. These findings represent a
shift in exogamy patterns for this group, particularly among
males. These changes may be linked to the larger number of
higher status Mexican Americans resulting from absolute occupation gains made by this group during the 1970s. It is specu-
lated that minority men benefited more than women from these
slight occupational gains. As a result, Mexican American men in
the 1970s may no longer have been as segregated from the dominant group, thus, increasing their likelihood to form personal
relationships and intermarry with dominant group females. Further research should examine how factors such as residential
patterns, occupation, income, education, and ethnic identity
maintenance influence outmarriage among Mexican American males
and females.

165. Valdez A ; Camarillo A ; Almaguer T. **The state of Chicano
research on family, labor and migration studies.** Stanford, California, Stanford Center for Chicano Research. 1983. 244 p.

Attention was given to the social class structure and role
content of **Mexican** American families and the values that reinforce the system of mutual support by extended family members.
Support system components were described as multidimensional,
multipurpose, and buttressed by an explicit set of culturally
derived expectations which are mediated by various demographic
factors, especially acculturation and social class. Though
cultural behaviors which typify the interactional patterns within many Mexican American households were reviewed, the authors
emphasized the great variety of means of familial adaptation.
The paper concludes with the presentation of a comprehensive
research model for understanding the Mexican American family.
This model details the factors normally considered in the literature as stressors and relates them within a temporal framework
that recognizes the importance of life changes and life events
as integral etiologic factors and processes in family life.

4. Sexual Activity

Of all of the categories of fertility determinants among Hispanics in the United States, least is known about their sexual activity. The few studies which have measured **proportion sexually active, age at first intercourse and interval between first intercourse and marriage** suggest that Mexican women may be older than whites or blacks when they initiate sexual activity, and may be more likely to delay sex until marriage. Preliminary studies of Mexican origin adolescents suggest that young women who have been in the U.S. longest are most likely to be premaritally sexually active. However, much more work is needed on this topic.

166. *Charnowski KM. Adolescent sexuality, contraceptive and fertility decisions. Chicago, Illinois, University of Chicago. 1982.

The research undertaken in this dissertation examines four aspects of sexuality, contraceptive, and fertility behavior for an urban sample of 496 adolescent females. The data set used for the analysis are the Chicago Urban League Young Chicagoans Study conducted in 1979 throughout the city of Chicago. The general results suggest racial differences for many of the dependent variables: the entrance into sexual activity, the occurrence of pregnancy in the sexually active subsample, and the selection of hypothetical pregnancy outcomes.

167. Darrow WW. Venereal infections in three ethnic groups in Sacramento. **American Journal of Public Health.** 1976 May;66(5): 446-50.

Blacks treated in Sacramento County, California clinics were most likely to have gonorrhea. Chicanos (**Mexicans**) were slightly more likely to have nonspecific urethritis and other sexually transmitted diseases, and whites were most likely to be uninfected. Whites tended to name greater numbers of different sexual partners, but differences among the three groups were not statistically significant. Among those who experienced symptoms, black men tended to delay significantly longer than Chicano men, and Chicano men tended to delay longer than white men. No differences in delays were found for women who reported symptoms. Black men more frequently reported to clinics with genitourinary symptoms and delayed significantly longer before seeking treatment. Future research should assess the relative contributions of sexual and health behaviors to the distribution of different sexually transmitted diseases in different groups.

168. *Golden JS ; Golden M ; Price S ; Heinrich A. The sexual problems of family planning clinic patients as viewed by the patients and the staff. **Family Planning Perspectives.** 1977 Jan/Feb;9(1):25-9.

A three part study conducted from October 1974 to February 1975 at a Los Angeles family planning clinic found that about 40% of the patients had sexual problems with which they needed help, but only one percent of the staff said they had seen as many as 20 patients with sexual problems. The patients were generally poor, young (31% under age 20, and 56% 20 to 30 years), white, and low parity. Forty-one percent were non-Latin white, 27% Latin, and 30% black. All three groups had similar sexual problems: 35% had difficulty achieving orgasm, 23% had pain with intercourse; no interest in sex, no feeling, and painful vaginal spasms each constituted 10 to 11%. The women also reported male problems with premature ejaculation accounting for 43%, difficulty in keeping an erection 18%, and too much interest in sex 20%. Two-fifths of staff members do not routinely ask patients questions related to sex, largely because of time pressure. Staff also mistakenly assumed that younger, Latin, unmarried, and less educated women have more problems when the facts are that all women have similar problems.

169. U.S. Department of Health and Human Services, National Center for Health Statistics. Marriage and first intercourse, marital dissolution, and remarriage: United States, 1982. By: Bacharach CA and Horn MC. **Advance Data.** 1985 Apr;107. 8 p.

This report presents data on the timing of first sexual intercourse in relation to first marriage, and the timing of marital dissolution and remarriage among ever married women in the United States. The findings of the report are based on preliminary data from the National Survey of Family Growth, Cycle III, conducted in 1982. About two-thirds of ever married women 15 to 44 years of age had had sexual intercourse before marriage. About 20% of all ever married women married within one year of initiating sexual activity, 23% married within one to three years, and about 25% married three or more years after their first intercourse. The statistics show that women of Hispanic origin were more likely than other women to delay their first sexual intercourse until marriage. No significant differences in cumulative rates of marital disruption between Hispanic and non-Hispanic women were found. Differences in remarriage rates between Hispanic and non-Hispanic women were not statistically significant.

PART TWO

PREGNANCY AND FERTILITY

1. Pregnancy and Prenatal Care

Although medical studies of prenatal and obstetrical care are only tangentially related to the purpose of this bibliography, **rates of pregnancy** are certainly relevant, as are particular barriers to the use of prenatal care which may account for negative birth outcomes for Hispanic women.

A number of authors have reported language and staffing barriers which might be expected to keep Hispanic women from utilizing prenatal services. Some studies suggest that foreign born Hispanic women and women born in Puerto Rico are less likely to come for **prenatal care** and more likely than non-Hispanics to begin care late. Despite this, the infants of Hispanic women appear to be at decreased risk of **low birthweight**, perhaps because of less maternal smoking. It is not clear whether this birth weight advantage holds for adolescent mothers as well. The one study which examines adolescent prenatal **risk behavior** found that Hispanic (Mexican) and Anglo teens were equally likely to smoke cigarettes or marijuana or to consume alcohol during pregnancy.

170. *Auerbach S ; Nathan B ; O'Hare D ; Benedicto M. Impact of ethnicity. **Society.** 1985 Nov/Dec;23(1):38-40.

This is a study of 172 teens under age 15 who registered for prenatal care at an MIC clinic in New York City between 1980 and 1982. This sample of medically indigent young women was 59% Hispanic (**Puerto Rican**) and 49% black. The authors report that girls from both groups were similarly likely to be in school at pregnancy or to leave while pregnant, but the blacks were much more likely to subsequently return (no tabular data are presented). This may be related to living situation since unlike the Hispanics, the young black mothers rarely married. The authors suggest that the Hispanic family, on both sides, is more likely to welcome the pregnancy. Blacks were also more likely to return to MIC for family planning and to select a reliable method of birth control.

171.   *Bristow C ; Cohn MR ; Huling T ; Soloway RD. **Services for sexually active, pregnant, and parenting adolescents in New York City: planning for the future.** New York City, Center for Public Advocacy Research. 1982. 120 p.

This is the first of a two volume report which documents and analyzes the findings of a study commissioned by the Center for Public Advocacy Research.   This volume provides an overview of adolescent sexual activity, pregnancy, and parenting in New York City,   including a demographic database for the City and its local jurisdictions; a description of the service needs of the population; an inventory of existing services; an analysis of the funding supporting these services; the identification of general programmatic and geographic gaps and duplications in service; and finally, conclusions and recommendations to help funders and planners maximize the impact of their resources on those adolescents who are pregnant, parenting or at risk of pregnancy and childbearing.   Hispanic data of interest include tables of pregnancy, birth, out-of-wedlock birth and abortion rates by age for young women in New York City from 1976 to 1980.

172.   Cadena MA ; Trevino MC. Utilization barriers to mater-nal/child health care programs of the urban, low income, Mexican American family: implications for a national health policy. Presented at the 105th Annual Meeting of the American Public Health Association, Washington, D.C. November 1, 1977. (Unpub-lished) 20 p.

Two aspects of accessibility are examined: geographical and social.   The latter seems more relevant here: ethnicity and culture are crucial factors affecting provider/consumer behav-ior.   Data collected for this study allowed a comparison of levels of utilization at three major urban centers in the south-west: Dallas, San Antonio, and Albuquerque.   Comparing the percent of births without prenatal care for Anglos and **Mexican** Americans between Dallas and San Antonio for 1976 show ratios of 1:4.6 and 1:4 respectively, Anglo to Mexican American; in Berna-dillo County, New Mexico, the Mexican Americans had the lowest percent of births without prenatal care.   The staffing patterns of the centers contacted appear to show a correlation between staffing by Mexican American providers to levels of utilization by Mexican American consumers.   While staffing patterns may reflect a degree of sensitivity to the ethnocultural composition and needs of the community being served, insufficient data was a limiting factor in developing a conclusive determination of correlation.   The data from the three centers clearly show that where the health care delivery system's socio-organizational structure reflects the ethnocultural structure of the community it serves, the distribution of health care is more evenly shared by its population.

173.   *Doyle MB ; Widhalm MV. Midwifing the adolescents at Lincoln Hospital's teenage clinics. **Journal of Nurse/Midwifery.** 1979 Jul/Aug;24(4):27-32.

This is a report of the first two years of care provided for adolescents in an evening prenatal clinic at Lincoln Medical Center in the South Bronx, New York. The attendees, from 12 to 19 years of age, were 70% Hispanic and 28% black.   They repre-sent approximately 20% of all teenagers who gave birth at Lincoln between 1975 and 1977.   Staffing was minimal: one obstetrician/gynecologist, two midwives, one nurse's aide, and

one clerk.   Emphasis was placed on education, good nutrition,
and continuity of care via midwifery caseloads.   Ninety-three
percent of the teenagers returned for six or more prenatal
visits.   Success, based on data from 204 delivered mothers, was
evidenced by the following: average maternal weight gains,
which improved from 21 (1976) to 28 pounds (1977); newborn
weights increasing from six pounds, 13 ounces to seven pounds,
13 ounces, and a decrease in low birth weights from 18 to six
percent.

174. *Moss N.   Individual deficits or social environment? Effects of social network members on risk behavior in adolescent
pregnancy. Paper presented at the American Public Health Association Annual Meeting, Montreal, Canada. (Unpublished) 1982. 3
p.

The data are derived from a one year hypothesis generating study
of adolescent pregnancy in San Jose, California.   Intensive
interviews were utilized to obtain information.   There were no
differences between Anglo and Hispanic teenagers in substance
use or timing of behavior change.   Most of those interviewed
knew that substance use is harmful to babies and acted on the
knowledge.   Anglo and Hispanic teens were about equally likely
to have used different substances at some time, depending on
financial resources. Almost every adolescent named at least one
person who was very helpful during pregnancy, and of these 47%
named their mother first.   The partner is the second key support
person, particularly early in pregnancy.   The mother and other
female relatives are particularly important for obtaining prenatal care.   In San Jose, there is a tendency for Hispanics to
tell partners and mothers about the pregnancy and to obtain
prenatal care more rapidly than do Anglos.   Those who received
information from their primary support person obtained care
faster than those who received only tangible help or emotional
support.   Intrafamilial communication may be more important than
tangible assistance in promoting early prenatal care for adolescents.

175. *Salazar SA.   Raza women and reproductive health issues.
In: **Hispanic report on families and youth.** Washington, D.C.,
National Coalition of Hispanic Mental Health and Human Services
Organizations. 1980. p. 37-41.

This paper advocates action which will give Raza (**Mexican**) women
choices regarding their reproductive functions and health.   It
focuses on teenage pregnancy, informed consent, sterilization
abuse and medical experimentation.   Pregnancy among most Raza
adult women is a high risk undertaking.   The risks are com-
pounded for teenage women who become pregnant.   In 1974, there
were one million pregnancies among women aged 15 to 19.   Fourteen percent resulted in miscarriages.   Babies born to teenage
mothers are two to three times more likely to die in the first
year than babies born to women in their 20s. The maternal death
risk is 60% higher for teens than for women over 20 years of
age.   Seven in ten teen mothers receive no prenatal care in the
first three months of pregnancy, and almost a quarter receive no
prenatal care at all.   Lack of access to care is a primary
problem.   Much of the abuse regarding reproductive care occurs
in the area of informed consent which requires educating the
patient and reeducating the medical profession.   Sterilization
abuse impacts severely on minority and poor women.   Racism,
poverty, lack of information, and absence of adequate government

sponsored measures to regulate abusive medical practices all play a part. Minority women in the United States have been subjected to medical experimentation to an unknown extent.

176. *U.S. Department of Health and Human Services, National Center for Health Statistics. Reproductive impairments among currently married couples: United States, 1976. By: Mosher WD. **Advance Data.** 1979;55:1-11.

Preliminary estimates, based on Cycle II of the National Survey of Family Growth conducted in 1975 by the National Center for Health Statistics, are provided for fecundity impairments, or involuntary conditions that make it difficult or impossible to have additional children, among currently married couples in the United States. Fecundity classifications included: 1) contraceptively sterile; 2) non-contraceptively sterile; 3) long interval (three years without contraception or pregnancy); and 4) subfecund (difficulty in carrying a pregnancy to term). Findings indicate that in 1976 about 6.9 million couples, or 25% of all married couples with the wife of childbearing age, had fecundity impairments, with most couples having one child or more and not wanting additional children. A significant minority of couples with impaired fecundity (about 2.7 million) wanted to have a baby or another baby, with about 848,000 of these couples childless and 688,000 with only one child. In all, couples with impaired fecundity who wanted to have a baby made up about ten percent of the married couples with the wife of childbearing age.

177. Ventura SJ ; Taffel SM. Childbearing characteristics of United States and foreign born Hispanic mothers. **Public Health Reports.** 1985 Nov/Dec;100(6):647-52.

This study compares maternal and infant health and sociodemographic characteristics of United States and foreign born Hispanic mothers and their babies, using data from National Vital Statistics and the 1980 National Natality Survey. While nearly half of all Hispanic, **Mexican** and **Puerto Rican** mothers were born in the U.S., fewer than ten percent of **Cuban** and other Hispanic mothers were U.S. born. Compared with foreign (**Central American, South American**) or Puerto Rican born Hispanic mothers, U.S. born mothers tend to be younger, less likely to have received delayed or no prenatal care, have higher educational attainment, and are more likely to be unmarried. The incidence of low birth weight among births to Hispanic mothers is relatively low. When the proportions of low birth weight are examined by nativity status, it is seen that births to foreign or Puerto Rican born women are consistently less likely to be of low birth weight. In an effort to account for these findings, mother's smoking status before and during pregnancy is examined. Compared with non-Hispanic mothers, Hispanic mothers are much less likely to have smoked before or during pregnancy. These data are examined to see if they account for the better outcome as measured by birth weight for Hispanic births, especially those to foreign or Puerto Rican born women.

178. *Wittenberg CK. Summary of market research for healthy mothers, healthy babies campaign. **Public Health Report.** 1983 Jul/Aug;98(4):356-9.

This paper reports the results of a market survey for the "Healthy Mothers, Healthy Babies" campaign conducted by the Los

Angeles Department of Health and Human Services.   All 137 participants met the following selection criteria: 15 to 34   years
old; black or **Mexican** American; currently pregnant or planning
to be in the next two years; had resided in the area for at
least two years; had never worked in a health related field; and
if Mexican American, spoke only Spanish or spoke Spanish at home
in preference to English.   All of the women were of low socioeconomic status.   The Mexican Americans complained that there
were too few Spanish speaking staff members in clinics.   Limited
Spanish language programming made television less effective with
Mexican Americans than with blacks.   Many teenage Mexican Americans listen to black oriented radio stations and to other English language radio stations rather than to those that broadcast
in Spanish.   Although only 36% of the Mexican American women
spoke Spanish exclusively, almost 90% of those from Los Angeles
and 66% of those from Chicago preferred to speak and read in
Spanish.   Many Mexican American women, because they do not want
to be regarded as backward or not Americanized, reject breast
feeding, which they associate with traditional Mexican practices.

2. Abortion

Many persons presume that Hispanic women will be less likely than non-Hispanics to undergo induced abortions because they are predominantly Catholic. Although reliable data on abortions are difficult to obtain for women of any ethnicity, available statistics suggest that Hispanic women may not be more reluctant than non-Hispanics to elect abortions.

Legal abortion ratios (abortions per 100 known pregnancies), like other fertility-related measures, are likely to vary considerably by Hispanic origin group. In New York City the ratios for Hispanic women (predominantly Puerto Ricans) are higher than those for blacks or whites. Data from the 1979 United States/Mexico border survey show a similar prevalence for Anglo and Mexican American women. However, Hispanic women aged 17 to 24 in the 1982 National Longitudinal Survey (predominantly Mexicans), report fewer abortions than do the whites.

179. *Anonymous. Fall in New York City abortions in 1975 is credited to birth control. **Family Planning Perspectives.** 1977 Jan/Feb;9(1):33.

For the first time since New York State legalized abortion in 1970, the number of abortions to New York City residents declined; in 1975 residents obtained 81,426 abortions, 4,472 fewer than in 1974. Abortions to non-residents dropped by 31%, presumably because of improved access in other communities since the 1973 Supreme Court decision. Births also continued to decline. The decline in pregnancies (abortions plus births) declined among all age groups except girls 17 and under. Fifty-one percent of abortions were to non-whites, a 1% decline; 35% to non-Puerto Rican whites, a 12% decline; and 14% to **Puerto Ricans,** a 2% decline. Number of abortions performed in the first trimester increased from 86% in 1974 to 89% in 1975. More than half were performed in free standing clinics. In 1969 there were 24 deaths reported due to illegal abortions in New York City. No illegal abortion deaths have been reported since 1973. Deaths following legal abortion declined from 12 in 1970-

71 to four in 1974-75.   1976 abortion figures are not yet available.

180.   Archdiocese of New York. Hispanics in New York: religious, cultural and social experiences.   Office of Pastoral Research. 1982.

This is a study commissioned by the Archdiocese of New York concerning church going, religiosity and attitudes toward sexual morality and social responsibility.   Respondents were Hispanic (**Puerto Rican**) men and women in New York City and a second sample of Hispanics from Rockland County.   The survey included questions on the acceptability of abortion, artificial contraception, premarital sex, and marital fidelity.   Comparing the responses between the Rockland County study, 64% of the Latinos believed firmly that abortion is always wrong, while 63% of the church goers in Rockland, and 32% of the non-church goers found it immoral.   As the Latino respondents grew in age, the tendency was toward a larger proportion believing that abortion is wrong. Over half of all Latinos felt that artificial contraception is wrong.   Of the total responses from the Hispanic study, 67% believe firmly that premarital sexual relations is wrong as compared with 61% of church goers, and only 18% of non-church goers in Rockland County.   Overall, 88% of all Latinos expressed a firm belief that married persons should have sexual relations only with their spouses.

181.   Aviaro H. Latina attitudes towards abortion. **Nuestro.** 1981 Aug/Sep;5(6):43-4.

This essay is based on interviews with 120 **Mexican** women in East Los Angeles.   Generally, there seemed to be three types of opinions toward abortion.   One group of women stated strong and unwavering opposition to abortion.   These women opposed abortion under all conditions, even when the pregnancy would endanger the mother's life.   Another group of women strongly supported abortion rights and tended to approve of abortions under all possible situations.   Finally, a third group of women, who represented the majority of those interviewed, had responses which reflected a more middle-of-the-road stand.   Most women approved or disapproved of abortion, depending on the reason for which the woman wanted to have one.   An overwhelming majority of women approved of abortion if it endangered the mother's life, if the fetus was abnormal, or in cases of rape or incest.   Similar opinions have been expressed by Anglos in nationwide polls.

182.   Bragonier JR ; Lowe EW.   The experience of two county hospitals in implementation of therapeutic abortion. **Clinical Obstetrics and Gynecology.** 1971;14(4):1237-42.

A study of the patterns of utilization and accompanying logistical problems of the Santa Clara Valley Medical Center and the Harbor General Hospital in California in trying to provide the necessary abortion services for their county's medically indigent is presented.   Both hospitals service a predominance of minority patients (Spanish Americans at Santa Clara, Spanish Americans and blacks at Harbor General in Los Angeles County). At Santa Clara the abortion rate has increased from 69 per 1,000 live births in 1968 to 370 per 1,000 in 1970.   While 58% of all live births there are Spanish American, only 16% of the abortions performed were on Spanish American women.   Because of the limited space at Harbor General, a counseling session is held at that hospital to encourage the patient to seek another facility for the abortion.   If the patient still requires public assistance, every attempt is made to admit her for the abortion.   To better serve the medically indigent, it is concluded that solutions must be sought to the problems of lack of abortion information in the community, lack of adequate facilities for the operations, and the latent staff antagonism toward abortion patients.

183. Fisher-Burton N. Abortion: a study of the perceptions of sixty abortion applicants and twenty service givers in Denver, Colorado. Doctoral Dissertation, University of Denver. 1976. 429 p. DAI;37(5-A):3184.

Feelings and attitudes of applicants about abortion as a solution, preabortion experiences in decision-making (including problem sharing with significant others), and applicant reactions to community services and delivery systems were studied in a sample of economically disadvantaged clients from two urban hospital clinics.   The clinics provided different social service systems, one using a group educational approach to orientation and the other using individual counseling.   Seventy percent of the clients found the preabortion experience very stressful, with many dwelling on destruction of life or other moral/religious concerns.   Ethnic minorities (Hispanic and black), and those classified as Catholic differed significantly from other clients in this respect.   No significant difference in satisfaction with the service delivery systems of the two clinics was found.   Together with their service givers, applicants recognized and verbalized the need for an adequate individual counseling system.   Even though applicants shared their decision-making problems with significant others, they felt alone with the situation.   Variables of age, education, ethnicity, and religion only rarely influenced the overall response patterns.   Findings supported selected components of crisis and decision-making theory.

184. *Gold EM ; Erhardt CL ; Jacobziner H ; Nelson FG. Therapeutic abortions in New York City: a twenty year review. **American Journal of Public Health.** 1965 Jul;55(7):964-72.

An examination of two decades (1943-62) of therapeutic abortions in New York City indicates that the frequency of therapeutic abortions has decreased substantially in that time period.   Differences between ethnic groups as well as those between hospital categories, both in gross incidence of therapeutic abortions and in frequency of individual indications, are apparently determined in part by general community attitudes, by the relative economics of the patients, and by their cultural and social mores.   The most important factors are probably the attitude of individual doctors and hospitals toward abortions.   Whites have more than five times the abortions of non-whites and 26 times that of **Puerto Ricans.**   The trend is downward for all three ethnic groups.   There is a much higher mortality rate among non-white and Puerto Rican patients arising out of abortions than there is among whites.   These results indicate the need for equalization of the opportunities for therapeutic abortions.   A constructive control program has two facets: 1) the New York State abortion law requirement that current community opinion and advances in scientific knowledge be reviewed often;   and 2) development of effective family planning programs as the most practical approach.

185. *Harris D ; O.Hare D ;   Pakter J ; Nelson FG. Legal abortion 1970-1971: the New York City experience. **American Journal of Public Health.** 1973 May;63(5):409-18.

This study of experience in New York City under the liberalized New York State abortion law during the first year of its operation (July 1, 1970 to June 30, 1971) derived its information mainly from certificates of termination of pregnancy required by the New York City Health Code. Among City residents who received abortion services; 43% were non-white and 10% were **Puerto Rican.**   For this same period of time and by way of comparison, 31% of all live births were non-white and 18% Puerto Rican. Among non-residents who had abortions performed, 90% were white, 9.5% were non-white and only 0.5% were Puerto Rican.   The much higher proportion of white non-residents reflects in part the financial problems for non-residents since they would need funds for travel as well as the wherewithal for the costs of abortion. This would tend to eliminate the deprived minorities lacking finances. In comparing the data for the first and second halves of this 12 month period, it appears that the proportion of non-white and Puerto Rican women of all residents who received services had increased.   A slight, but perceptible increase was also noted among non-residents in the number of minority groups seeking abortions.

186. *Kramer MJ. Legal abortion among New York City residents: an analysis according to socioeconomic and demographic characteristics. **Family Planning Perspectives.** 1975 May/Jun:7(3):128-37.

The social, economic and demographic characteristics associated with abortion procedures are discussed.   The sample population consisted of 1.7 million women 15 to 44 years of age in New York City between September 1970 and August 1971.   By juxtaposing vital records of the New York City Department of Health with United States Census Bureau summary statistics, age adjusted rates of legal abortion are computed by race for each of 296 resident areas within the City.   It was found that women were obtaining legal abortions at a rate equivalent to 1.2 procedures over the reproductive span and that the abortion rate for blacks and **Puerto Ricans** doubled that for whites.   Moreover, legal abortion was utilized most among women from low income areas and among areas where education is low and where only a small percentage of school age children attend parochial schools.   But, it was only because blacks were concentrated at the low income, low education, low labor force participation end of the spectrum that the neighborhood pattern of abortion rates showed the mentioned trends.

187. *Ortiz CG. Teenage pregnancy: factors affecting the decision to carry or terminate pregnancy among Puerto Rican teenagers. Doctoral Dissertation, University of Massachusetts. 1982. 127 p. DAI;43(8-A):2559.

This exploratory study examined the variations in the degree of influence that family relationships, religion, education, and income had on the decision to carry or abort pregnancy.   A non-random sample of 43 pregnant **Puerto Rican** teenagers, (21 who carried and 22 who aborted), were interviewed while waiting for health services in various clinics in New York City during the spring of 1982.   As hypothesized, girls in the carry group were more influenced and supported by family and friends than those

in the abort group.   Fathers were the least influential persons
in both groups, while mothers were the most influential in the
carry group and sisters in the abort group.   Brothers, boy-
friends, and best friends were more influential for carry girls
than for abort girls.   The carry and abort groups were significantly different according to comparisons in the degree of
religious devotion. Girls in the abort group reported a greater
degree of religiosity for themselves and their families than
those in the carry group. Furthermore, girls who received strong
support from family and friends reported a higher degree of
satisfaction with their decision than those less supported.
Finally, girls in the abort group were more likely to continue
their education than those in the carry group.   Although the
girls came from poverty levels, higher family incomes were
reported by the abort group.

188. *Pakter J ; Harris D ; Nelson F. Surveillance of abortion
programs in New York City. **Bulletin of the New York Academy of
Medicine.** 1971 Aug;47(8):853-74.

This article reviews the first six months' experience in New
York City with the liberalized abortion law of July 1970.   The
law, which permits abortions upon request up to week 24 of
gestation without residency restriction, made it essential for
the Health Department to incorporate protective standards into
the New York Health Code (Article 42, Abortion Services) such
that any pregnancy over 12 weeks may only be terminated in a
hospital. Of the 43,959 abortions performed, 56% were performed
on non-residents.   Ethnic distribution among residents was 50%
white, 41% black, and 9% **Puerto Rican**. Among the non-residents
it was over 90% white and less than 9% black or Puerto Rican.
Sixteen percent of the resident patients and 26% of the non-
residents were teenagers. Seventy-five percent of all abortions
were performed at week 12 or earlier, usually by suction curettage.   The leading complication in early terminations was per-
foration of the uterus (3%), while the incidence of complications after week 12 of gestation was much higher, including
retained placenta (10%) and infection (9%).   Six deaths resulted
from legal abortions during this period.   One conclusion is that
pediatricians should provide more counseling for young patients
to curb the rise of unwanted and out-of-wedlock pregnancies.

189. *Pakter J ; Nelson F. Abortion in New York City: the first
nine months. **Family Planning Perspectives.** 1971 Jul;3(3):5-12.

An analysis of New York City's experience in providing approximately 47,000 abortions in the first nine months (July 1, 1970
to March 31, 1971) after the state's liberalized abortion law
went into effect shows that safe prompt terminations of pregnancy can be performed upon women of all socioeconomic groups.
The morbidity rate was 6% for abortions under 12 weeks and 28%
for those over 12 weeks. Hospital admissions for septic abortions and illegitimate births decreased to the lowest point
since such data have been recorded.   The ratio of total abortions per 1,000 live births was 422 for whites, 594 for non-
whites, and 258 for **Puerto Ricans**. Puerto Rican women accounted
for 10% of abortions, considerably lower than their proportion
of live births; 18%. The ratio of abortions to live births was
considerably higher for New York City black women than it was
for white or Puerto Rican women.   Whereas for black women the
ratio was about six abortions for every ten live births, for
white women the ratio was four abortions for each ten live

births, and the ratio was less than three abortions for each ten live births among Puerto Rican women.   The data indicate that women have sought and obtained abortions earlier in pregnancy and abortion mortality rates have markedly decreased.

190. *Pakter J ; Nelson F. A study of repeaters of abortions. Paper presented at the 103rd Annual Meeting of the American Public Health Association, Chicago, Illinois. (Unpublished) November 19, 1975. 48 p.

Since the inception of legalized abortions in New York City in July 1970, there has occurred a definite increase in the number and percentage of New York residents who have had repeat abortions.   Abortions increased from 69,711 to 85,590 between 1972 and 1974.   The number of women having repeat abortions for this same period increased from 14% to 22%.   The increase in the number of repeaters exceeded the increase in the number of women undergoing a first abortion.   In order to further assess this trend, certificates were reviewed for the period 1972 to 1974 and information collected on the characteristics of women having repeat abortions as well as those having first abortions.   Among the non-white repeaters, teens were in higher proportion than among the whites, followed by the **Puerto Ricans**; the range was 12% for non-white teen repeaters, 11% for whites and 10% for Puerto Ricans.   The proportion of non-white repeaters rose from 46% in 1972 to 54% in 1974, while for the Puerto Ricans it rose from 10% in 1972 to 14% in 1974, and for the whites the proportion dropped from 44% in 1972 to 32% in 1974.   In 1974, among the multiple repeaters, the non-whites accounted for more than one-half (52%), the whites for about one-third (33%), and the Puerto Ricans for about 15%.   The Puerto Rican repeaters were most likely to have had a previous live birth or births and the white repeaters the least likely to have had previous births. The Puerto Rican repeaters showed marked increases in numbers for each parity group.   The white repeaters, seconded by the Puerto Ricans had the highest proportion of early terminations.

191. *Pakter J ; O'.Hare D ; Nelson F ; Svigir M. Two years experience in New York City with the liberalized abortion law: progress and problems. **American Journal of Public Health.** 1973 Jun;63(6):524-35.

The New York City Department of Health from July 1, 1970 to June 30, 1973, collected pertinent data on the liberalized abortion law for New York City.   Approximately two-thirds of the 334,865 abortions reported were for non-residents.   For dilation and curettage (D&C), and saline the greatest number was in proprietary hospitals.   The suction method accounted for 64% of all methods, with an increase from 56% to 70% in the second year. The greatest proportion seeking abortion was in the 20 to 29 age group.   Teenagers accounted for 29% in the first year, 34% in the second year for non-residents and 17% and 18% respectively for residents.   Among residents receiving abortions, 45% were non-white, 44% white and 11% **Puerto Rican** for the two years combined.   The ratio of abortions to live births in 1971 was 411 per 1,000.   There was an 12% decline in births and a 12% drop in out-of-wedlock births from 1970-71.   The infant mortality rate declined to 21 per 1,000 live births in 1971 and to 20 in 1972. Among residents the ratio of abortions to live births was about 400 per 1,000 with the highest ratio (563 per 1,000) for non-whites and lowest (250 per 1,000) for Puerto Ricans. Whites were intermediate at 373 per 1,000.

192. *Poliak J ; Morgenthau JE. Adolescent aborters: factors associated with gestational age. **New York State Journal of Medicine.** 1982 Feb;82(2):176-9.

The study objective was to determine if the medical and counseling program provided by the Family Life Education Program (FLEP) at the Mount Sinai Adolescent Health Center in New York City was associated with the timing of pregnancy interruption. FLEP offers a comprehensive program of sex education, contraception, gynecologic care, pregnancy diagnosis, and counseling to unmarried teenage residents of East Harlem. The medical records of 113 patients were examined. Teenagers in the 13 to 16 age group (58%) were significantly more likely to terminate pregnancy after 11 weeks than the 17 to 20 age groups (35%). The teenagers in the late abortion group were no more likely to be black or Hispanic than the early abortion group, and no group was more likely to be on Medicaid or self-paying than the other. There was a positive correlation between gestational age at abortion and previous enrollment in FLEP. Almost twice as many early as late aborters had been FLEP enrollees. Teenagers aborting after 11 weeks were significantly more likely to have never used any form of contraception than were those aborting early. Late aborters (47%) showed nearly a threefold greater incidence of poor school performance over early aborters (17%).

193. *Steinhoff PG. Background characteristics of abortion patients. In: Osofsky HW and Osofsky JD, eds. **The abortion experience: psychological and medical impact.**   Hagerstown, Maryland, Harper and Row. 1973. p. 206-31.

Any survey of characteristics of women seeking abortion must take into account the population served by the facility as a whole, the community attitudes, and the availability of abortion to various racial and ethnic groups. Unlike other countries, where most abortion users are over age 30, in the United States women under 25 are disproportionately likely to obtain abortions. Abortion rates for never married women are almost double those for married women. Abortion is seldom used for spacing. Gold et al. found that in 1960-62, the rate of therapeutic abortions per 1,000 live births was five times as high among whites as among non-whites. The white rate was 26 times as high as the Puerto Rican rate. Pakter and Nelson report that between July 1970 and March 1971 the rate of abortions per 1,000 live births in New York City was 422 for white women, 594 for non-white women, and 258 for Puerto Rican women. The consistently lower rate of abortion among Puerto Ricans in New York City, both before and after legalization, may be due to cultural attitudes which make abortion a less likely option for the pregnant woman.

194. *Tietze C ; Lewit S. Abortion. **Scientific American.** 1969 Jan;220(1):21-7.

In the modern world abortion is the most widespread means of fertility control. In the United States, one of the restrictive countries of the world, 235 deaths from abortion were listed in 1965. In another study cited, of the deaths from complications of pregnancy and childbirth, abortion accounted for 25% of the deaths of white women, 49% of the non-white women, and 56% of the **Puerto Rican** women in New York City from 1960 to 1962. In countries that have allowed legal abortion such as Denmark, Sweden, Japan, Hungary, Czechoslovakia, and Romania, birthrates have declined as abortion rates increase.

3. Fertility

The best data on current and cumulative fertility to women of different ethnic origins come from vital statistics and from the census. These are supplemented by special surveys with fertility variables such as the Current Population Survey, the National Survey of Family Growth, the Survey of Income and Education, and the National Longitudinal Survey.

Hispanic women aged 18 to 44 (predominantly Mexican Americans) have higher **fertility rates** than either black or white women in the United States. They begin childbearing early, have a rapid pace of **subsequent births,** and therefore, large **completed family size.** The differences in fertility among the various Hispanic groups are also quite pronounced. Mexican women have the highest rates, and Cuban women have the lowest.

During the 1970s in the U.S. women of all ethnic groups experienced a decline in general fertility and a decline in **unwanted births.** These decreases were particularly rapid for Hispanic and black women, although they continue to have higher rates of unwanted fertility than white women.

Much less data are available regarding the fertility of Hispanic adolescents in the U.S. From census data and vital statistics we do know that their birth rates fall between those of white and black adolescents, but sampling error precludes reliable calculation of trends in Hispanic adolescent fertility over time.

195. Alba F. La fecundidad entre los Mexicano Americanos en relacion a los cambiantes patrones reproductivos en Mexico y los Estados Unidos. (Fertility among Mexican Americans in relation to the changing reproductive patterns in Mexico and the United States). **Demografia y Economia.** 1982;16/2(50):236-49.

This study includes a comparison of fertility levels of **Mexican** Americans with those of Mexicans and of Americans, and an analysis of differential fertility patterns in the three populations.

Mexican American fertility is higher than that of the general United States white population and similar to that of the Mexican population, but data permitting exact comparisons are lacking. In 1969, Mexican American women aged 35 to 44 had an average of four children, while U.S. women the same age had three. However, Mexican American fertility has been declining in the past few decades; in 1950 it was 100% greater than white American fertility, while by 1970 it was only 45% greater. Changes in the fertility patterns of Mexican Americans from 1950-70 appear to have paralleled those of the U.S. population, with increases from 1950-60 and decreases from 1960-70. Available information also suggests that Mexican American fertility varies by educational status in approximately the same form as does that of U.S. white fertility, with fertility negatively related to education. Fertility differentials between Mexican Americans and the white U.S. population decline by over 50% when education is held constant. Data on recent fertility behavior in Mexico show the same negative association between education and fertility, with the total fertility rate six for those with incomplete primary education and four or less for those with more education.

196. Alvirez D ; Bean FD ; Williams D. Patterns of changes and continuity in the Mexican American family. In: Mindel CH and Haberstein RW, eds. **Ethnic families in America: patterns and variations** (second edition). New York, Elsevier North-Holland. 1981. p. 269-93.

The authors illustrate the importance of analyzing the ethnic factor in understanding family life styles. **Mexican** Americans constitute one of the largest ethnic groups in America. Certain cultural patterns that have been thought to carry great weight in family life among Mexican Americans do not in actuality uniformly characterize their family patterns. The most noticeable feature of the Mexican American family is its size relative to other groups of Americans. The fertility of Mexican Americans is substantially higher than other groups. Census materials on children born show that the fertility of the Mexican American population, compared with the total white population, has been high and remains so, and that their fertility is as high or higher than the black population. However, as the authors indicate, the traditional Mexican family structure has been influenced by the forces of urbanization, female labor force participation, and geographical and social mobility.

197. *Bachu A ; O'Connell M. Developing current fertility indicators for foreign born women from the Current Population Survey. **Review of Public Data Use.** 1984 Oct;12(3):185-95.

This paper presents fertility estimates for foreign born women from the April 1983 Current Population Survey (CPS). The survey data indicate that women 18 to 44 years old from Latin America, especially from Mexico, have a higher fertility rate than their European counterparts, with women from Asia having an intermediate level of fertility. Data are included for **Cubans** and **Mexicans.** In addition, the childbearing of Latin American women made up about one-half of the estimated 271,000 children born to all foreign born women in the year preceding the April 1983 CPS. An evaluation of the data indicates that although the survey information is useful in identifying fertility differences among foreign born women in the United States, the relatively large sampling errors associated with these data restrict their use-

fulness for detecting annual changes in the childbearing patterns of immigrant women.

198. Bean FD ; Bradshaw BS. Mexican American fertility. In:
Teller CH, Estrada LF, Hernandez J, and Alvirez D, eds. **Cuantos
somos: a demographic study of the Mexican American population**.
Austin, Texas, University of Texas, Center for Mexican American
Studies. 1977. (Mexican American Monograph No. 2).

The relatively high fertility of the **Mexican** American population
has been extensively documented and often discussed, but the
question of whether the fertility of that population remains
high and unchanging over time has not been adequately addressed.
This paper examines trends in Mexican American fertility in
comparison to Anglo American fertility from 1950 to 1970 in the
southwestern states, and notes some of the socioeconomic characteristics, practices, and attitudes which may support the relatively high rate of reproduction of this population. In
focusing upon trends in fertility, attention is devoted primarily to cumulative fertility (as expressed by the average number
of children ever born to women of certain ages) rather than
current fertility, since the former measure is the only one
available for all the time periods and areas studied.

199. Bean FD ; Stephen EH ; Opitz W. A demographic profile of
the Mexican American population in the United States. Austin,
Texas, University of Texas, Texas Population Research Center.
1984. 15 p. (Texas Population Research Center Paper No. 6.024).

The authors attempt to provide a demographic profile of the
Mexican origin population in the United States. Problems of
definition are first considered. Attention is then given to
population size and distribution; age and sex distribution;
fertility; family and marital status; mortality; and labor force
participation, occupations, and income. As assessed by the data
from the 1980 Census, perhaps the most distinguishing feature of
this population has been its extremely rapid rate of growth
during the 1970s. While most of this increase could be attributed to the high fertility generally characteristic of Mexican
origin women, a substantial part of it was also due to the
influx and the counting in the 1980 Census of undocumented
migrants from Mexico. Over a million such persons have been
estimated to have been residing in the U.S. in 1980. It is
impossible to know whether this group represents a smaller large
fraction of the total number of undocumented immigrants from
Mexico in the country. Second, an overriding demographic
feature of the Mexican origin population is its generally disadvantaged socioeconomic status. In general, the socioeconomic
characteristics of the Mexican origin population imply a socioeconomic position intermediate to that of blacks and Anglos.

200. *Bradshaw BS ; Bean FD. Some aspects of the fertility of
Mexican Americans. In: Westoff CF and Parke R Jr, eds. **Demogra-
phic and social aspects of population growth**. Washington, D.C.,
U.S. Government Printing Office. 1972. p. 139-64. (Commission on
Population Growth and the American Future, Research Reports,
Vol. 1).

The purposes of this report are: 1) to bring attention to some
of the circumstances, practices, and attitudes among **Mexican**
Americans which may support their relatively high reproduction
rate as a group; and 2) to note some of the factors which lead

some Mexican American couples to have larger or smaller families than others.   Historical records, published and unpublished Bureau of the Census tabulations, and the results from a study of 348 Mexican American couples in Austin, Texas, are drawn upon.   Mexican American fertility, as measured by ratios of children ever born per 1,000 women, remains much higher than the fertility of other white women, and may continue to be somewhat higher than fertility of black women.   Slightly lower age at marriage of Mexican American women probably has a small positive influence on fertility, but this effect may be offset by a negative effect from lower proportions marrying and slightly more widowhood and separation.   The limited data available suggest that contraceptive use may be emerging as an important variable affecting fertility.   The numbers of children wanted by husbands and wives in the survey of couples is about 4.4 on the average. These desires for many children are evidently supported by, and are congruent with, a generally positive attitude toward large families.

201. *Bradshaw BS ; Bean FD. Trends in the fertility of Mexican Americans: 1950-1970. **Social Science Quarterly.** 1973 Mar;53(4): 688-96.

This paper examines trends in **Mexican** American fertility from 1950 to 1970 in the southwestern states.   By 1950, the first year for which fertility data based on the Mexican American population beyond the second generation is available, the number of children ever born to Spanish surnamed women 15 to 44 years of age averaged 54% more than the number born to non-Spanish surnamed women in the southwest.   By 1960, however, the gap between non-Spanish surnamed women and Mexican American and Spanish surnamed women was reduced to 35%.   The convergence may be explained by the more rapid rise in Anglo than in Mexican American fertility in that period.   Differences between Mexican American and Anglo American fertility emerge much more sharply after an adjustment for age composition is made.   In general, Mexican Americans and Anglo Americans in the southwest have followed similar trends in fertility since 1950.   The average fertility of women in both groups was higher in 1960 than in 1950, especially for women under 35 in 1960.   Comparable declines in fertility in both groups occurred by 1970.   Period fluctuations have not been as sharp among Mexican Americans as among Anglo Americans.

202. *Darabi KF ; Ortiz V. Childbearing Among Young Latino Women in the United States. **American Journal of Public Health.** (Forthcoming) 1986.

In this paper the authors compare rates of ' early childbearing among white, black, **Mexican** and **Puerto Rican** young women, and observe how these rates compare after controlling for marital, socioeconomic, and generational statuses.   Perhaps the most notable finding is the marked difference in fertility behavior between Mexican and Puerto Rican adolescents.   In some ways Puerto Rican women appear to be more similar to non-Hispanic blacks than to Mexicans or Anglos.   Although they have lower current fertility than black women, like blacks, Puerto Ricans are more likely to bear their first child outside of marriage. A second parallel is that among both Puerto Ricans and blacks the likelihood of a premarital first birth was inversely related to socioeconomic status.   In contrast to the Puerto Rican and other adolescents, the Mexicans are an anomaly.   Their rates of marital first births are double those of the Puerto Ricans, and their rates of premarital first births are notably low at the lowest socioeconomic level.   The Mexican/Anglo differences in marital and premarital fertility that persist within socioeconomic categories are consistent with the subcultural differences theory that explain ethnic differences in adult marital fertility.

203. Davis C ; Haub C ; Willette J.   United States Hispanics: changing the face of America. **Population Bulletin.** 1983 Jun;38 (3). 44 p.

An analysis of demographic trends among the Hispanic (**Mexican, Puerto Rican, Cuban**) population of the United States is presented using data from various sources,   including the 1980 U.S. Census.   A definition of the term Hispanic is first presented. The Hispanic population is then described with regard to age and sex composition,   residence,   fertility,   mortality,   family and marital status, education, employment and occupation, and income and poverty.   Consideration is also given to both legal and illegal immigration and to future projections of the size of this population. With relatively high fertility and growing legal and illegal immigration,   the U.S. Hispanic population increased by some 265% from an estimated four million in 1950 to 14.6 million and 6.4% of the total population counted in the 1980 census. By 2020, they could number some 47 million and displace blacks as the largest U.S. minority if immigration were to continue at the recent estimated level of one million a year (legal plus illegal, Hispanics plus all others). Self-identified as persons who trace their heritage to Spanish speaking countries, Hispanics consist of Mexican Americans (60% of the total),   still concentrated in the southwest; Puerto Ricans living mainly in New York and New Jersey; Cubans headquartered in Florida; and the second largest,   more scattered "other Hispanic" group from some 16 other Latin American countries and Spain,   plus some Mexican Americans established many generations in the U.S. southwest.

204. Jaffe AJ ; Cullen RM ; Boswell TD. The changing demography of Spanish Americans. **Studies in Population.** New York City, Academic Press. 1980. xiii, 426 p.

The authors present an analysis of the demographic and fertility characteristics,   along with summary economic traits,   for five Spanish origin groups living in the United States.   The groups are defined as Hispanic (**Mexican, Puerto Rican, Cuban, Central American,** and **South American**). The analysis is presented in two parts.   In the first part,   the authors describe the theoretical aspects of the study and broad findings that pertain to all the Spanish origin people who live in the U.S.   The second part consists of separate chapters for each of the five groups analyzed.   The extent to which Hispanics are merging into the U.S. population as a whole is considered,   and the primary variables affecting that convergence are identified. Data are from the 1970 U.S. Census.   Thirty pages of statistical tables are included.   These tables include highest year of school completed, children ever born, labor force participation,   median earnings and selected characteristics of women.

205. Juarez RZ. Collection of Mexican origin vital and health statistics in south Texas counties along the United States/ Mexico border. Paper presented at the 20th National Meeting of

the United States Public Health Conference on Records and Statistics, Washington, D.C. August 13-15, 1985.

The purpose of this paper is to identify: 1) progress in the collection of Hispanic vital and health statistics, with a specific focus on the population of **Mexican** origin; 2) some problems that still persist; and 3) some suggestions for addressing these problems.   Data were obtained from a visual examination of 623 birth certificates and 504 death certificates selected from three registrar offices in two United States/Mexico border counties in Texas, and from information gathered by an Hispanic National Committee on Vital and Health Statistics supported by the Ford Foundation in 1983.   The author emphasizes the need to maximize the appropriate use of the ethnic identifiers if Hispanic vital and health statistics are to become a reality in some states. Furthermore, self-identification of the appropriate ethnic origin is necessary as rates of structural assimilation increase.

206. *Mann ES ; Salvo JJ. Characteristics of new Hispanic immigrants to New York City: a comparison of Puerto Rican and non-Puerto Rican Hispanics. Paper presented at the Population Association of America Annual Meeting, Minneapolis, Minnesota. (Unpublished) May 3-5, 1984. 49 p.

Up until the 1966-70 period, most Hispanics coming into New York City were migrants of **Puerto Rican** origin or descent.   Since 1970, however, the tide of Puerto Rican immigration has subsided and immigration of non-Puerto Rican Hispanics has increased. Although classified under the Hispanic cultural banner, these newer non-Puerto Rican immigrants come from a variety of cultural and socioeconomic backgrounds, all quite different from that of Puerto Ricans.   Using Summary Tape Files 2 and 4 of the 1980 Census, and the Public Use Micro Data Samples, this research provides a comprehensive look at the demographic and socioeconomic characteristics of Puerto Ricans and "other Hispanics," those non-Puerto Rican immigrants exclusive of Cubans and Mexicans, in New York City.   The results show wide differences in socioeconomic status of the groups, closely related to basic disparities in fertility, labor force participation and most of all, family structure and composition. Moreover, an examination of the two largest "other Hispanic" subgroups, **Colombians** and **Dominicans**, revealed differences which were, in many instances, wider than those between Puerto Ricans and all "other Hispanics."

207. Mosher WD ; Hendershot GE. Religious affiliation and the fertility of married couples. **Journal of Marriage and the Family.** 1984 Aug;46(4):671-7.

Using the 1973 and 1976 National Survey of Family Growth (nationally representative samples totalling 14,000 married women), the authors present a wide range of national estimates of the fertility of married couples in religious groups in the United States.   Hispanic Catholic couples had the highest number of wanted pregnancies per woman (2.35), followed by white Catholics (2.21), and white and black Protestants (2.05 and 2.06).   The smallest religious groups (Jewish, other, and none), all had substantially lower fertility than Protestant and Catholic couples.   White wives with no religious affiliation had the lowest mean number of children even born (1.29), the smallest number of total births expected (1.96), and the lowest number of wanted

pregnancies per woman (1.36).   Jewish couples also had substantially lower fertility than Protestant and Catholic couples.
These results seem to support a minority status hypothesis,
i.e., that minority group status reduces fertility, except among
groups that have a pronatalist ideology and norms discouraging
the use of efficient contraceptives.

208. *Mott FL. Evaluation of fertility data and preliminary
analytical results from the 1983 (fifth round) survey of the
National Longitudinal Survey of Work Experience of Youth. Ohio
State University, Center for Human Resources Research. 1985.

The fifth round survey of the National Longitudinal Survey of
Work Experience of Youth in 1983 included interviews with 6,143
male and 6,078 female respondents who were between the ages of
18 and 26 when interviewed during the first half of 1983.   The
interviews with the men updated the complete live birth histories and related data collected in the 1982 survey round.
The interviews with the women updated from 1982 the pregnancy
histories and related records of maternal and infant health and
child care.   A major objective of these analyses which focus on
early school leaving and fertility, early parity progression,
and fertility expectations, is to clarify issues relating to the
quality of those data and to convey to other researchers some of
the unique aspects of this longitudinal data set.   Hispanic and
white young women are much less likely than blacks to have a
birth before graduating from high school.   However, Hispanics
who do get pregnant have the lowered probabilities of school
completion.

209. *Mott FL. Fertility related data in the 1982 National
Longitudinal Survey of Work Experience of Youth: an evaluation
of data quality and some preliminary analytical results. Ohio
State University, Center for Human Resource Research. December
1983. 148 p.

This report evaluates the quality of the fertility related data
in the 1982 round of the National Longitudinal Survey of Work
Experience of Youth and summarizes highlights of findings from
these fertility data. The report specifies the potential magnitude of reporting errors, how these potential error levels are
related to characteristics of the respondents, and the procedures used to clean up the fertility records.   The analytical
sections of the report examine differentials in period and
cohort birth rates, sexual activity and contraception, birth
wantedness, and pregnancy outcome for selected respondent characteristics within cross-tabular and multivariate frameworks.
Characteristics considered include race and ethnicity (white,
black and Hispanic), religion, education, various aspects of
family stability, social class, and geographic residence. The
multivariate results suggest the utility of a variety of background factors and more proximate respondent attitudes and
behaviors for investigating a variety of adolescent and young
adult fertility-related attitudes and behavior.

210. *New York City Department of Health, Bureau of Health Statistics and Analysis. Summary of vital statistics: 1979, 1980,
1981, 1982, the City of New York.

These papers present a summary of vital statistics for the
population of New York City during the given year.   Fertility
related statistics presented in the tables include percentages

of total births of certain characteristics such as low birth
weight, late or no prenatal care to teenagers, and out-of-
wedlock mothers by Health Center District of residence, infant
mortality by ethnic group, incidence of abortion and spontaneous
terminations by age and residence of mother, and live births by
mother's age and descent or origin (including **Mexican**, **Puerto**
Rican, **Cuban** and other Hispanic). The summaries also include
deaths by cause, chief causes of death, age adjusted death
rates, cases of reportable diseases, and life expectation
tables.

211. *O'Connell M ; Rogers CC. Differential fertility in the
United States: 1976-1980. **Family Planning Perspectives.** 1982
Sep/Oct;14(5):281-6.

The United States fertility rate rose slightly, from 67 births
per 1,000 women aged 18 to 44 in 1976 to 71 per 1,000 in 1980,
according to the Current Population Surveys (CPS) for those
years. The most notable increases occurred among women who were
30 or older, married women living with their husbands, women
living in the south, and women whose family income was at least
$25,000. One-third of women 18 to 44 years old who had a child
in the year preceding the June 1980 CPS were employed at the
time of the survey. This finding reflects the rapid return of
women to work after a birth. Twenty percent of the mothers were
living in poverty areas, and 27% were living in families with
incomes less than $10,000. Forty-five percent of all women who
had a birth between July 1979 and June 1980 were high school
graduates. Women who were not high school graduates accounted
for 25% of all births, while college graduates accounted for
another 13%. Almost half of the births to college graduates
were first births, indicative of delayed childbearing among this
group of women. Hispanic women, although constituting less than
7% of women 18 to 44 in 1980 accounted for ten percent of all
births. Their fertility rate of 107 births per 1,000 women was
50% higher than the rate for all women.

212. Rindfuss RR. Fertility and migration: the case of Puerto
Rico. Madison, Wisconsin, University of Wisconsin, Institute for
Research on Poverty. June, 1975. 25 p. (Institute for Research
on Poverty Discussion Paper No. 280-75).

This paper is an examination of the relationship between migration and fertility, using measures of current fertility and
cumulative fertility. By combining records from the United
States Census with records from the **Puerto Rican** Census it is
possible, for the first time, to compare the fertility levels of
Puerto Ricans who migrated to the U.S. with those of their
counterparts who remained in Puerto Rico. In general, the
effect of migration to the mainland is to reduce fertility, but
this reduction is very small. Furthermore, there is some evidence that this effect of migration on fertility has been dimin-
ishing.

213. *Slesinger DP ; Okada Y. Fertility patterns of Hispanic
migrant workers in Wisconsin. Paper presented at the 52nd Annual
Meeting of the Population Association of America, Pittsburgh,
Pennsylvania. (Unpublished) April 14-16, 1983. 20 p.

The childbearing history and family planning practices of women
in migrant farmworker families in Wisconsin were analyzed. The
migrant farmworker population in Wisconsin is over 90% Hispanic

(**Mexican**), with approximately half of the workers born in Mexico and half born in the United States.   In the summer of 1978, a survey of migrant farmworkers in Wisconsin was conducted.   About one-third of the migrant women in the childbearing years were 15 to 29 years old; 30% were in their 30s; and 37% were in their 40s.   The average number of births to date was 4.3.   Migrant women who spoke only Spanish had borne one more child, on the average, than women who were bilingual (5.3 compared to four). Age was found to be related to the number of live births, yet, when age was statistically controlled, education appeared to be even stronger in explaining the variation in number of live births and expected completed family size.   There was some evidence that younger women have obtained more education than the older women, but even for younger women, relatively few had completed high school.   Thus, to date, little difference in fertility behavior between the older and younger cohorts was observed.   Over one-third of the women both under and over 30 had their first birth at age 18 or younger.

214. *Spencer G. The contributions of childlessness and non-marriage to racial and ethnic differences in American fertility. Paper presented at the Population Association of America Annual Meeting. (Unpublished) April 9-12, 1980. 25 p.

The degree to which fertility differentials between whites and blacks, and whites and women of Spanish origin, are due to differences in childlessness among ever married women and among single women, and varying proportions of ever married women, is examined for 1970 and 1978.   The fertility differential between blacks and whites aged 18 to 44 would have been considerably greater if the proportion of ever married among blacks the same as among whites, and would have been smaller if black women had the white level of childlessness, especially among single women.   Simultaneous control of variations in childlessness and proportions ever married did not affect the 1970 fertility differential, but would narrow it by 13% in 1978.   The differ-ential between whites and women of Spanish origin would be 19% smaller in 1970 and 52% smaller in 1978, if white levels of childlessness had been met.   The fertility differential was not changed very much between these groups when proportions of ever married were obviated.   The net effect of controlling for these variables among whites and women of Spanish origin was to reduce the fertility differential by 17% in 1970 and 55% in 1978.

215. Sweet JA. Comparisons of own children marital fertility estimates using 1970 decennial census, 1976 Survey of Income and Education, and 1970 and 1976 Current Population Survey data. Madison, Wisconsin, University of Wisconsin, Center for Demo-graphy and Ecology. 1981. 22 p. (Working Paper No. 81-34).

This paper investigates the comparability of three data sets: the decennial Census; the 1976 Survey of Income and Education (SIE); and the March 1976 Current Population Survey (CPS). Com-parisons are made separately for the white, black, and **Mexican** American populations.   Only the 1976 estimates can be compared for Mexican American women since the Mexican American population is not separately identified prior to 1972.   In 1976 the CPS estimate is 9% higher than the SIE estimate (520 versus 471). The Census/SIE and CPS estimates are not interchangeable.   The Census and SIE are reasonably comparable.   The CPS estimates are consistently higher than the Census and SIE series, particu-larly for blacks and Mexican Americans.   In sum, the Census/SIE series provides reasonable trend estimates, but differentials among subgroups are not valid.

216. Sweet JA. Differentials in the rate of fertility decline: 1960-1970. **Family Planning Perspectives.** 1974 Spring;6(2):103-7.

Data in this article are taken from the 1960 and 1970 Census of Population which includes the household composition along with age of each member. Measure of fertility was the average number of children under age three living in the same household with their own mother, married and under age 40.   This approximates the number of births a woman has had in the past three years by looking at the number of children under age of three living with her in the household, and, in the same way, can identify the number of births each woman had in a previous year from number of children under age one living with her.   Shortcomings to this method are listed. Fertility declines have been more rapid during 1957-60 and 1967-70 among blacks, American Indians and **Mexican** Americans (groups which previously had the highest fertility) than among urban whites.   Data are also summarized for **Puerto Rican,** urban and rural, Japanese and Chinese Americans. Among urban whites, fertility decline has been heavily concentrated among those of low income.   The decline was particularly rapid for third and higher order births, indicating a possible concentration of completed fertility in two child families. The rapid decline, and the narrowing of traditional fertility differentials among various subgroups, has important implications in the areas of poverty, education, and the role of women in society.

217. *Torres A. Hispanic adolescents: focus on fertility. Presented·at the 112th Annual Meeting of the American Public Health Association, Anaheim, California. (Unpublished) November 11-15, 1984. 20 p.

The primary data sources were the National Center for Health Statistics reports on births in 1980, the Census Bureau's Current Population Surveys, and a 1979 survey of contraceptive use among women of childbearing ages in the United States/Mexican border states carried out by the Centers for Disease Control. Of the 53 millon U.S. women of reproductive age in 1980, 3.6 million were of Hispanic origin. Nearly 780,000 of the Hispanic women aged 15 to 44 were teenagers.   In 1980 there were about 307,200 births to Hispanics in 22 states reporting Hispanic percentage.   About 58,000 or 19% of these births were to women under age 20.   Among the different Hispanic ethnic groups, **Puerto Ricans** had the highest percentage of adolescent births to women under 18:   43% compared with 39% among **Mexican** Americans, 35% among **South Americans** and **Central Americans,** and 29% of **Cubans.**   Forty-three percent of all births to Hispanic women under age 20 were out-of-wedlock.   The rate of out-of-wedlock childbearing among Hispanics aged 15 to 19 was about 40 per 1,000.   Forty-one percent of currently married women of Mexican origin aged 15 to 19 and seven percent of never married women 15 to 19 were using contraception at the time of the survey.

218. *Torres A. Information on fertility patterns: focus on Hispanic adolescents. Paper prepared for the Alan Guttmacher Institute, New York City, (Unpublished) 1981. 47 p.

In 1980, fertility among United States adolescents of Hispanic origin was consistently higher than among white adolescents.

Fertility among black women was higher than for either white or Hispanic women. Among all adolescents of Hispanic origin, **Mexican** Americans had the highest birth rate.   These differences in fertility among race and ethnic groups persist in the U.S./Mexican border states.   While one-third of all births among whites are out-of-wedlock, 43% of births to adolescents of Hispanic origin were out-of-wedlock and 86% of all births among blacks were out-of-wedlock.   Among Hispanics, **Puerto Ricans** showed a greater   likelihood   toward out-of-wedlock births.   The study showed that 41% of currently married women of Mexican origin aged 15 to 19 were using some form of contraception at the time of the survey.   The proportion increased sharply to 71% among women aged 20 to 24, remained stable until aged 35 to 39, and then fell to 48% at ages 40 to 44.   Anglos were more likely to use the condom and diaphragm and less likely to use the pill or the IUD than were Mexican Americans.   Among all adolescents of Hispanic origin, Mexican Americans had the highest birth rate, 96 per 1,000 and **Cubans** the lowest, 25.   Puerto Ricans showed a birth rate of 83 and other Hispanics, 52.

219. *Tyrer LB. Poverty, family planning, and health. **Planned Parenthood Review.** 1984 Winter;3(4):11-2.

Fertility rates in the United States are highest among poor, minority, and non-working women.   Although the fertility rate is 71 per 1,000 women aged 18 to 44 years, the rate is 130 per 1,000 among women not in the labor force, 84 per 1,000 among blacks, 107 per 1,000 among Hispanics, and 94 per 1,000 among women with family incomes of $5,000 per year.   Moreover,   these groups of women who are at greatest risk of pregnancy are generally at greatest risk of an adverse outcome of pregnancy, suggesting a need for fertility regulation services directed toward these groups.   Poor women and younger women are either less likely to use contraception or are more likely to experience contraceptive failure.   In addition, if abortion services were more available to poor women, especially welfare recipients, the incidence of unwanted, high risk pregnancies would be significantly reduced.   Women must be assured the knowledge and means to exercise control over their own fertility.

220. *U.S. Department of Commerce, Bureau of the Census. Fertility of American women: June 1980. Current Population Reports (CPR), Population Characteristics. 1982 Oct;P-20(375):1-89; and ---, Fertility of American women: June 1981. CPR, Population Characteristics. 1983 Apr;P-20(378):1-63; and ---, Fertility of American women: June 1982. CPR, Population Characteristics. 1984 Apr;P-20(387):1-67; and ---, Fertility of American women: June 1983. CPR, Population Characteristics. 1984 Nov;P-20(395):1-63; and ---, Fertility of American women: June 1984. CPR, Population Characteristics. 1985 Nov;P-20(401).

These reports present statistics on the actual and expected fertility rates of American women based on data collected in the June Current Population Surveys.   Statistics on birth expectations, current fertility patterns, premarital first births, and socioeconomic differences in childbearing are discussed.   The fertility rates of women of Spanish origin are compared with those of non-Hispanic women.

221. U.S. Department of Commerce, Bureau of the Census. Persons of Spanish origin in the United States: March 1980, advance report. Current Population Reports (CPR), Population Character-

istics. 1981 May;P-20(361); and ---, Persons of Spanish origin in the United States: March 1982. CPR, Population Characteristics. 1985 Jan;P-20(396). 80 p.; and ---, Persons of Spanish origin in the United States: March 1985, advance report. CPR, Population Characteristics. 1985 Dec;P-20(403).

These reports represent a continuation of the annual series of reports presenting demographic, social, and economic data on persons of Spanish origin residing in the United States. Most of the data shown were collected as a supplement to the Current Population Surveys (CPS) of the Bureau of the Census. Additional data from other CPS supplements are also included. This report includes data for the total Spanish origin population and its subcategories: **Mexican, Puerto Rican, Cuban, Central American** or **South American**, and other Spanish origin. Among the characteristics presented are age, marital status, education, voting and registration, fertility, employment, family composition and size, income, and poverty status. In addition to the data for the Hispanic origin population, data for the overall population and for persons not of Spanish origin are also shown in the report.

222. U.S. Department of Commerce, Bureau of the Census. Population Profile of the United States: 1979. Current Population Reports (CPR), Population Characteristics. 1980;P-20(350):1-52; and ---, Population Profile of the United States: 1980. CPR, Population Characteristics. 1981;P-20(363):1-56; and ---, Population Profile of the United States: 1981. CPR, Population Characteristics. 1982;P-20(374); and ---, Population Profile of the United States: 1982. CPR, Population Characteristics. 1983; P-23(130); and ---, Population Profile of the United States: 1983-1984. CPR, Population Characteristics. 1985 Sep;P-23(145).

These reports provide a statistical description of the social, economic, and demographic characteristics of the population of the United States in the given year. Most of the statistics in the report are estimates based on sample data from the Census Bureau's Current Population Survey. Information is included on the population of Spanish origin and its subcategories (**Mexican, Puerto Rican, Cuban, Central American, South American**, and other Spanish origin). Tables and graphs feature data on population growth, age, marital and family status, education, population distribution, employment, income, race, and Spanish origin.

223. *U.S. Department of Health and Human Services, Centers for Disease Control. Texas fertility: childbearing patterns and trends, summary 1950-1977. Atlanta, Georgia, Bureau of Epidemiology. 1980;29:950-77. (Family Planning Evaluation Division, No. 20.7011).

Fertility levels (births) in Texas have followed a pattern similar to fertility levels in the overall United States, although the general fertility rate (GFR) in Texas has been higher than the national GFR each year it has been examined since 1950. Fertility increased in the mid-1950s, then declined until 1969 when there began a two year increase. Rates were highest for white women with Spanish surnames, and intermediate for black women. Rates declined from 1970 to 1977 in all age and ethnic groups except white 15 through 19 year olds with Spanish surnames. Women 30 years of age or older had the lowest fertility rate, and women 20 to 24 years of age had the highest. White women with Spanish surnames had slightly higher rates of out-of-

wedlock births than those with non-Spanish surnames, and much
lower rates than black women.   In 1977, an estimated 16,740
unintended births occurred to white women with non-Spanish surnames and black women in Texas.   Unintended births to 15
through 19 year olds accounted for the vast majority of all
unintended births. Births to females younger than age 15 and to
married women who had previously borne three or more children
accounted for relatively few of the unintended births.

224. *U.S. Department of Health and Human Services, Centers for
Disease Control. United States/Mexico Border survey of maternal
and child health family planning: 1979, advanced report. Atlanta, Georgia, Family Planning Evaluation Division. 1980. 24 p.

In 1979 the Centers for Disease Control collected social, demographic, fertility, and contraceptive data from a sample of
2,135 women, aged 15 to 44, living in the United States/Mexican
border states of Texas, New Mexico, Arizona, and California.
Among the respondents, 37% were Anglo, 59% were Hispanic, and
four percent were black or other. Thirty-nine percent of the
Hispanics and 48% of the Anglos were 30 to 44 years of age.
Fifty-six percent of the Hispanics and 66% of the Anglos were
currently married. The Hispanic women, as a group, had less
education and lower family incomes than the Anglos.   The mean
number of children born to ever married women was 4.77 for the
Hispanics and 3.05 for the Anglos. Sixteen percent of the Hispanics and 12% of the Anglos said their last pregnancy was
unwanted.   The Hispanic women also reported a higher number of
unplanned pregnancies than the Anglos. Sixty percent of the
Anglos and 46% of the Hispanics were currently using contraception.   Sterilization and oral contraceptives were the most popular methods of contraception among both the Hispanic and the
Anglos, however, male sterilization was less common among the
Hispanics.

225. U.S. Department of Health and Human Services, National
Center for Health Statistics. Birth and fertility rates for
states, United States: 1980. By: Taffel S. **Vital and Health
Statistics.** Data from the National Vital Statistics System. 1984
Sep;21(42):1-31.

This report presents in tables 1980 birth and fertility rates
for the United States, divisions, and states. Birth data used
to compute rates are based on information obtained from the
birth certificates of the 50 states and the District of Columbia.   Birth and fertility rates for the U.S. and individual
states are based on the total resident populations of the respective areas.   The population data by race as enumerated in
the 1980 Census have been modified for this report to maintain
comparability with previous census and vital statistics data
series.   Since 1978, the birth certificates of a number of
states have requested information on parents' ethnic origin. It
was therefore possible to include birth and fertility rates for
the Hispanic population of the 22 states reporting this information in 1980.   These states accounted for an estimated 90% of
all births of Hispanic origin in the U.S. in that year. In the
comparison of birth and fertility rates by ethnic origin, births
are classified by the ethnic origin of the mother as reported on
the birth certificate.   In the 22 reporting states with 307,163
Hispanic births, the birth rate and fertility rate for this
group overall was 24 and 95 respectively. The **Mexican** subgroup
exhibited the highest fertility, followed by **Puerto Ricans,** with

the **Cubans** having the lowest rates.

226. *U.S. Department of Health and Human Services, National
Center for Health Statistics. Births of Hispanic parentage:
1979. By: Ventura SJ. **Monthly Vital Statistics Report.** 1982;31
(2-Supplement):1-11; and ---, Births of Hispanic parentage:
1980. By: Ventura SJ. **Monthly Vital Statistics Report.** 1983;32
(6-Supplement):1-18; and ---, Births of Hispanic parentage:
1981. By: Ventura SJ. **Monthly Vital Statistics Report.** 1984;33
(8-Supplement):1-16; and ---, Births of Hispanic parentage:
1982. By: Ventura SJ. **Monthly Vital Statistics Report.** 1985;34
(4-Supplement).

These papers provide information on births of Hispanic parentage
during the given year from those states reporting ethnic or
Spanish origin on birth certificates.   Statistics are presented
for birth and fertility rates, live birth order, age of mother,
birth weight of infant, educational attainment of mother, and
month prenatal care began, by Hispanic origin of mother (**Mexican, Puerto Rican, Cuban, Central American,** and **South American**),
and by race for non-Hispanic origin mothers.

227. U.S. Department of Health and Human Services, National
Center for Health Statistics. Socioeconomic differentials and
trends in the timing of births. By: Ford K. **Vital and Health
Statistics.** Data from the National Survey of Family Growth. 1981
Feb;23(6):1-49.

Included in this report is an analysis of cumulative birth
probabilities within first marriages in the United States.
Trends and differentials in these probabilities by race, Hispanic origin, education at first marriage, farm origin, religious preference, and timing of first births are discussed and
shown in table form.   Probabilities are shown for specified
birth order intervals and age at first marriage or previous
birth.   The data were collected in 1973 and demonstrates that a
woman's age at first marriage or her most recent birth is closely associated with how quickly the next birth will take place.
There were significant differences in the timing of births in
different racial, ethnic, and religious groups. Women of Hispanic origin were more likely to have their first birth within a
year of marriage than were other women; to have a second birth
within 18 months of the first; and to have a third birth within
18 months of the second.   Since the late 1950s there has been
some lengthening of birth intervals for the first two births and
declines in the probabilities of later births within first
marriages in the U.S., but there are still significant groups
who frequently have births at closely spaced intervals.

228. *Ventura SJ. Vital issues on vital records for Latinos.
Paper presented at the 113th Annual Meeting of the American Public Health Association, Washington, D.C. November 18, 1985. 7 p.

The Hispanic fertility rate in 1982 was 96 births per 1,000
women aged 15 to 44 years, 48% higher than the rate of 65 for
non-Hispanic women.   There are wide variations in fertility
among the various Hispanic groups and between white and black
women. **Mexican** women had the highest rate, 102 births per
1,000; followed by **Puerto Rican** women, 68; and **Cuban** women, 54.
The rate for white women was 64 and for black women it was 84.
Consistent with the higher fertility of Mexican, Puerto Rican,
and black non-Hispanic women is their tendency to begin child-

bearing at younger ages and to have larger families.   Teenage
mothers accounted for an average of 20% or more of Mexican,
Puerto Rican, and black non-Hispanic births, compared with about
ten percent of Cuban and white non-Hispanic births.   In addition, Mexican, Puerto Rican, and black non-Hispanic women were
about twice as likely to be having their fourth child or more as
were Cuban and white non-Hispanic mothers.   Hispanic mothers are
more than twice as likely as white non-Hispanic mothers and much
less likely than black non-Hispanic mothers to be unmarried.
Only 41% of Mexican mothers and 50% of Puerto Rican mothers had
completed high school, compared with 76% of Cuban mothers, 84%
of white non-Hispanic mothers, and 65% of black non-Hispanic
mothers.

229. Westoff CF. Planned and unplanned births in the United
States: the decline in unwanted fertility, 1971-1976. **Family
Planning Perspectives.** 1981 Mar/Apr;13(2):70-2.

This paper focuses on trends in unwanted fertility by comparing
rates derived from the 1973 and 1976 National Survey of Family
Growth.   Rates of unwanted fertility have been calculated based
on women at risk of unwanted childbearing, controlling for the
length of exposure to such risk.   Three indices are presented,
indicating what the experience would be in a hypothetical cohort
subject to the rates prevailing during the 30 months preceding
each survey.   There is clear evidence of a significant decline
in unwanted fertility during the first half of the 1970s.   For
married women, the chances of having an unwanted birth by 15
years since the last wanted birth declined from 0.21 in the
1971-73 period to 0.11 in the 1974-76 period.   The cumulative
number of unwanted births declined from 0.38 to 0.20 births per
woman.   This decline affected all subgroups (by race, Hispanic
origin, region, metropolitan status, education, income, and
religion), and was roughly equally distributed throughout the
social structure.   Differentials continued to persist, however,
with higher rates of unwanted fertility among blacks, Hispanics,
those least educated and most poor.

230. Whiteford LM. Family relations in Seco County: a case
study of social change. Doctoral Dissertation, Milwaukee, Wisconsin, University of Wisconsin. 1979. 207 p. DAI;41(5-A):2195.

Case studies of a limited number of families are presented to
describe and analyze changes in family structure among **Mexican**
Americans who are, or were, migrant farm workers.   The setting
is a rural town on the Mexico/United States border in Texas.
Work patterns, division of labor, patterns of communication
between husband and wife, and among women were investigated.
Changes in birth rates, patterns of family planning, economic
opportunities, and individual and familial aspirations are discussed.   Life histories, including health, migration, and work
histories were collected and are used as a baseline from which
to evaluate the changes presently occurring.   The smuggling of
drugs and guns, the presence of federally funded health, education and job programs, and the decrease of labor intensive
agriculture are considered in respect to their effect on familial economic strategies.

PART THREE

FERTILITY REGULATION

1. Family Planning Services and Clients

Data on the use of birth control methods and services by Hispanic adult women come basically from the National Survey of Family Growth, and, for the 1970s, from the now discontinued National Reporting System for Family Planning Services. From these sources it appears that Hispanic women are equally, or even more likely than black or white women to use **organized family planning services,** but less likely to seek these **services from private physicians.** A lower proportion of Hispanics than non-Hispanics are **current users of contraception,** probably because of higher family size desires and rates of current pregnancy among the former. Because of their higher fertility desires, fewer pregnancies to Hispanic women are classified as "unwanted"; therefore, when wantedness is included in measures of failure rates, Hispanic women have the lowest **cumulative contraceptive failure rates.**

Hispanic women on the United States/Mexican border were slightly more likely than Anglo women to have been surgically **sterilized** in the 1979 survey, but Mexican men were much less likely than Anglos to have had a **vasectomy.** In fact, this large Anglo/Mexican difference in vasectomies is not explained by differences between the ethnic groups in socioeconomic status, marital status, religion or number of childen.

Data on contraceptive use and clinic use among younger Hispanics are more difficult to obtain since there are very few Hispanic adolescents in the National Survey of Family Growth, and since they were not included in any of the waves of the National Survey of Young Women, from which most of our knowledge of adolescent contraceptive behavior is obtained for black and white young women. Statistics for some comparisons of contraceptive use and method choice come from reports of large adolescent clinical services in the northeast, the 1979 U.S./Mexico border survey, and the National Longitudinal Survey of Youth.

231. *Anonymous. Birth control: clinics as a major source of care for poor teenagers, and for more affluent. **Family Planning**

Perspectives. 1979 May/Jun;11(3):197-8.

The 1976 National Survey of Family Growth was examined by the Alan Guttmacher Institute against the enrollment statistics of the organized family planning program, conducted under the auspices of the Department of Health, Education and Welfare's National Center for Health Statistics. The data showed that 58% of all currently married fecund women made a medical visit for contraception in the three years before the survey, compared to 51% before 1973. Fifty-nine percent of white women made clinic visits in the three years previous to 1976 compared to 46% of black women and 51% of Hispanic women. Clinic attendance showed a seven percent increase among whites, while a two percent decrease occurred among blacks. Use of organized services was much more common among women below 150% of the poverty level which is $8,700 for a non-farm family of four. These observations indicate that due to the availability of organized clinic service, an increased number of poor, as well as non-poor United States married women obtained medical family planning care in the 1970s. Clinics were the major source of care for both poor teenagers and adolescents of a higher income level. Married teenagers were more likely than older married women of 25 to 44 years to have made a family planning visit to the clinic.

232. Atkinson DR ; Winzelberg A ; Holland A. Ethnicity, locus of control for family planning, and pregnancy counselor credibility. **Journal of Counseling Psychology.** 1985;2(3):417-21.

White (n=40) and **Mexican** American (n=40) women seeking counseling at a Planned Parenthood agency were randomly assigned to four counselor descriptions and then asked to rate the counselor's credibility and attractiveness. The four counselor descriptions varied the counselor's ethnicity (white vs. Mexican American) and philosophy regarding the locus of control for family planning (individual choice vs. family choice). No evidence was found that Mexican American or white women view ethnically similar counselors as more credible or attractive than ethnically dissimilar counselors. The hypothesis that white women would rate the counselor with an individual choice philosophy highest, whereas Mexican American women would rate this counselor lowest, was also unsupported. Mexican American women rated the counselor as more trustworthy (regardless of counselor ethnicity) than did Anglo American women.

233. Bonta D ; Kaplan C ; Waltman NM. Family planning needs of the Los Angeles Hispanic population. Paper presented at the 44th Annual Meeting of the United States/Mexico Border Health Association, Monterrey, Mexico. April 28-30, 1986.

The purpose of this paper is to assess the extent and the nature of the need for family planning services in the Hispanic population residing in Los Angeles County. Los Angeles Regional Family Planning Council, Inc. (LARFPC) coordinates the delivery of family planning services of 109 family planning sites in Los Angeles County. During the fiscal year 1984-85, LARFPC provided services to 153,732 women, approximately 51% reported to be of Hispanic descent. Hispanics are the fastest growing group in Los Angeles County. In 1980 they comprised 28% of the total population compared to just 18% in 1970. This increase is due to both the natural increase of the resident population and the continuing immigration. As a result, the Hispanic population constitutes 30% of the total 15 to 34 year old group of potential childbearers in Los Angeles. They accounted for 57% of the total adolescent births and 53% of births to mothers 14 or younger. These women have a higher risk of poor pregnancy outcome and greater socioeconomic disadvantage since early childbearing contributes to lower educational levels, and fewer job opportunities. Data for this study include state, county and private sources, in addition to information gathered through the LARFPC clinics. Indicators used to assess the need for family planning services included fertility and mortality rates, perinatal mortality, age distribution, income and education. Implications for reproductive health services geared to the Hispanic population and adolescents in particular are examined.

234. *Cressy MK. Factors related to the use of family planning services of low income teenage mothers. Doctoral Dissertation, New York City, Columbia University, Teachers College. 1976. 131 p. DAI;36(12-B):6072.

This article surveys factors related to the use of family planning services of low income teenage mothers during the first eight postpartum months. Two hundred and thirty-five low income teenage mothers who had delivered live infants in one of five metropolitan New York hospitals were interviewed in the hospital during their postpartum period. Their records were checked and a questionnaire sent to them eight months later to discover their status in reference to the use of family planning services. According to their records, 34% had not accepted family planning services; 35% had accepted at the six week postpartum examination, but had not returned as recommended during the seven months following the initiation of services; 32% had accepted at this time and returned for their follow-up appointment. A positive correlation was found between use of family planning services and the reported quality of prenatal clinic and labor and delivery room nurses, and the reported use of birth control by teenage acquaintances. Subjects were more likely to return for services when oral contraceptives or IUDs were prescribed than if diaphragm or foam were prescribed. Blacks and Protestants were more likely to return than **Puerto Ricans** and Catholics.

235. *Family Planning Council of New York City. **Family planning fact book of New York City: 1960-1973.** New York City, December, 1975. 122 p.

This is an update of the original fact book prepared by the Family Planning Council of New York City, 1973. It was hoped that the book would help in planning, evaluating, and improving family planning services in the City. Twenty-five tables plot the data and an introduction summarizes the accumulated data. There was a need to review the family planning situation because of changes in the population and changes in the abortion law in recent years. The percentage of whites declined and that of blacks and **Puerto Ricans** increased substantially in the years between 1940 and 1973. The number of high parity births has declined in recent years, due largely to increased use of family planning services. The general fertility rate in New York City declined from 82 per 1,000 eligible females in 1970 to 60 in 1973. By 1973 there were almost eight abortions performed for every ten babies born in the City. Infant mortality rates were down. The family planning program in the City largely serves the indigent, the ones who need it most. Nearly half the births in the City took place in subsidized hospitalizations, 27% were

out-of-wedlock, and 26% of the women giving birth had late or no
prenatal care.   Family planning information is now being provided in City schools.

236. *Jones JE ; Namerow PB ; Philliber SG. Reproductive health
care services for adolescents in a hospital based setting: a
four year report. New York City, Columbia University, Center for
Population and Family Health. 1983.

In the fall of 1977, Columbia Presbyterian Medical Center initiated specialized services for contraceptive care and counseling to young people aged 21 years and younger with the opening
of the Young Adult Clinic (YAC) by the Center for Population and
Family Health and the Obstetrics and Gynecology Service of
Presbyterian Hospital.   The clinic was designed and implemented
as part of the overall reorganization of the Ambulatory Ob/Gyn
Services for women in the Hospital's Vanderbilt Clinic.   This
report summarizes the first four years of the YAC service and
describes the characteristics of some 5,834 patients who made
17,864 visits between October 1977 and September 1981.   Tables
include data on background characteristics, histories, method
choice, pregnancy and revisits.   Hispanic clients were consistently more likely than blacks to first come to the clinic in
order to get a pregnancy test.

237. Marin BV ; Marin G ; Padilla AM. Attitudes and practices
of low income Hispanic contraceptors. Los Angeles, California,
University of California. 1981. 20 p. (Spanish Speaking Mental
Health Research Center, No. 13).

One hundred Hispanic (Mexican) women seeking family planning
services were interviewed about attitudes and practices in an
attempt to explain the higher fertility rate of Hispanic women.
The mean desired family size (3.34) was higher than that of
women nationally.   While children were considered very important, controlling family size was viewed as more important by
these women.   Regression analyses were used to predict both
present and desired number of children.   Age of the women and
age at the birth of the first child were the strongest predictors of fertility, followed by spouse's desired family size,
respondent's desired family size, and respondent's education.
Desired family size was most strongly predicted by partner's
desired family size, followed by age at the birth of the first
child, age of respondent, and birth in Latin America.   Being
born in Latin America was related to desiring a larger family
size.   Findings suggest the potential importance of the partner's attitudes on the woman's contraceptive behavior and the
influence of the acculturation process on desired family size.

238. Minkler D ; Looper T. Factors affecting family planning
services to non-English speaking immigrants. Advances in Planned
Parenthood. 1978;13(3/4):14-23.

Non-English speaking immigrants require special attention in the
planning and provision of family planning services.   In particular, attention to cultural as well as linguistic barriers to
care is necessary.   Knowledge of fertility-related beliefs and
practices on the part of the family planning service in the
country of origin; readiness to change health behavior patterns;
and prior exposure to family planning policies, education, and
services on the part of immigrants are of great value in tailor-
ing services to their special needs.   Experience with four

immigrant groups in San Francisco (Spanish speaking, Chinese, Korean, and Filipino) illustrates the use of bilingual staff and volunteers, decentralized facilities, integration of family planning with other health services, and special culturally compatible outreach programs that expand the usual health delivery network.

239. *Morgenthau JE ; Rao PS ; Thorton JC ; Cameron O. Adolescent contraceptors: follow-up study. **New York State Journal of Medicine.** 1977 May;77(6):928-31.

The contraceptive behavior of 421 women who attended the family life education program at an adolescent health center from April to October 1974 was followed by means of chart review through September 1975. Sixty-three percent of the patients continued to use a single method of contraception throughout their period of observation. This consistency was correlated with success rate. Significantly higher proportions of whites used the diaphragm (p<.05) and the Dalkon Shield (p<.05) as compared with blacks or Hispanics. In general, the younger Hispanics show a significantly (p<.01) higher usage of the Lippes Loop while the older blacks show the lowest usage. For the oral methods, non-whites exhibit a significantly higher proportion of use than whites (p<.01). Forty patients became pregnant during the study period while attempting contraception. Of these, about 70% of the total group, but only 50% of those under 18 years of age, chose to have abortions. Pregnancy rates were lowest among oral contraceptive and copper-7 users in a consideration of the entire cohort. The data suggest that successful contraceptors are those who tend to stay with a given method.

240. *Namerow PB ; Jones JE. Ethnic variation in adolescent use of a contraceptive service. **Journal of Adolescent Health Care.** 1982;3:165-72.

The purpose of this paper is to compare black, Hispanic (**Puerto Rican, Cuban**), and white teenagers' experience with a contraceptive service in New York City. Data are taken from information obtained from nearly 4,000 patients who made about 12,000 visits to the program during its first three years of operation. Patients' reasons for using the contraceptive facility, their visit patterns, clinic continuation rates, methods accepted, patterns of method utilization, as well as their pregnancy rates, and their intentions for pregnancy resolution are examined. Black patients had more clinic visits than did white and Hispanic patients, and their duration of program contact was the longest. Several method preference differences exist among the three ethnic groups. Pregnancy rates while in contact with the program were highest among black patients, followed by Hispanic and then white patients. Service delivery directions suggested by these findings are discussed.

241. *Namerow PB ; Kalmuss D ; Jones JE. An evaluation of the Young Adult Clinic: a six year report. New York City, Columbia University, Center for Population and Family Health. 1985. 26 p.

The Young Adult Clinic was initiated in 1977, in response to a community identified need for preventive health services for adolescents. About two out of five patients are of Hispanic origin, slightly more than half are black and the remainder are white or of other ethnic origin. Paralleling the change in the ethnic composition of the neighborhood in which the Young Adult

Clinic is located, the proportion of Hispanic patients increased from 33% during the first two years of the program to 42% during the fifth and sixth program years.   The Hispanics differ from the blacks on several measures.   They are less likely to have had sex by age 13, and more likely to postpone first sexual experience to age 17 or later.   Blacks have the longest intervals (14.1 months) between first sexual experience and first clinic visit, followed by Hispanics (13.5 months), and then whites (12.6 months).   However, Hispanic patients are substantially less likely to report that they came to the clinic for a birth control method than are black or white teens, and Hispanics are more likely to come to the clinic for a pregnancy test than are black or white teenagers.

242.   *Namerow PB ;   Philliber SG. Reproductive health care services ·for adolescents in a hospital based setting: a four year report.   New York City,   Columbia University, Center for Population and Family Health. 1982. 18 p.

In the fall of 1977, the Columbia Presbyterian Medical Center in New York City began specialized services for contraceptive care and counseling to young people aged 21 years and younger with the opening of the Young Adult Clinic by the Center for Population and Family Health.   In the years 1972-80, the number of live births in the community which surrounds the center increased by 33%, while all other areas experienced declines.   The number of clients with previous pregnancies and the proportions who initially come to the clinic for pregnancy testing are high.   Ultimately, the prime objective of a teen contraceptive program is the prevention of an unintended pregnancy.   There is no single reliable way to estimate pregnancies among the program's patients.   However, of those who initially came to obtain a contraceptive, 14% returned for a second visit with a positive pregnancy test.   Although the estimate cannot be immediately interpreted as either "clinic" pregnancy rates, or as pregnancy rates among adolescents in the area around the Medical Center, it is useful because it may bracket the actual pregnancy rates among clinic patients.

243.   *Okada LM ; Gillespie DG. Effect of public family planning on unwanted pregnancies.   Paper presented at the 104th Annual Meeting of the American Public Health Association, Miami Beach, Florida. October 17-21, 1976. 14 p.

A sample of 10,193 women were interviewed between August and November of 1972 in seven areas with varying ethnic and economic compositions.   The effect of two types of family planning resources are examined: public family planning resources and private family planning resources.   It was learned that the use of a family planning resource greatly increased contraceptive effectiveness.   Large numbers of unwanted pregnancies occurred among women using contraception before they became associated with a family planning resource.   The cumulative failure rate at the 12th month of an interval in the before period was 25% among women who subsequently went to a public family planning resource, compared with 35% among women who later went to a private family planning resource.   The influence of income on the cumulative failure rates is unclear.   The cumulative failure rates for the pregnancy intervals before resource use was highest for the whites, followed by blacks, and was lowest among the Spanish women.   The cumulative failure rates were particularly high in the before period for all groups of women under 25 years of age, regardless of birth order or whether they subsequently used a public or private family planning resource.

244. *Philliber SG ; Jones JE. Staffing a contraceptive service for adolescents: the importance of sex, race, and age. **Public Health Report.** 1982 Mar/Apr;97(2):165-9.

Other studies have suggested that the composition of clinic staff is important in attracting and maintaining contact with adolescents seeking contraceptive services.   In this paper the importance of age, sex, and ethnicity of counselors and medical providers is examined. Female clients of the Young Adult Clinic at Columbia Presbyterian Hospital, New York City (most of them low income blacks or Hispanics), were asked to complete ques-tionnaires. The 150 respondents, aged 16 to 21 years, indicated that the sex of the counselor and examiner was more important to female teenagers than ethnicity or age.   Clinic administrators seeking to provide contraceptive services to teenagers should make an effort to include at least one female counselor and medical provider.   However, none of these characteristics was very important to the majority of patients.   These findings are discussed in the context of the literature on the provision of contraceptive services to teenagers and on patient preferences for counselors or therapists in general.

245. *Philliber SG ; Namerow PB ; Jones JE. Age variation in use of a contraceptive service by adolescents. **Public Health Reports.** 1985 Jan/Feb;100(1):34-40.

This study examined contraceptive use and pregnancy patterns among four groups of a total of 4,318 adolescents: 14 years and younger; 15 to 17 years; 18 to 19 years; and 20 to 21 years. The percentage of Hispanic adolescents in these groups was 36%, 39%, 38%, and 46% respectively. The data were collected during more than 7,000 visits to an adolescent contraceptive clinic made by the adolescents over a five year period.   When compared to the black adolescents, Hispanic young women were more likely to give pregnancy test as a reason for first visit to the clinic.   They were less likely to come back for a revisit at 12 months or later, or to have ever used pills or IUDs. Among the women who accepted contraceptive methods, Hispanics were less likely than blacks to be consistent users. These differences were confirmed in multivariate analyses after controlling for differences in background characteristics.   Despite this, the black patients were more likely to be pregnant at a subsequent visit.

246. *Ralph N ; Edgington A. An evaluation of an adolescent family·planning program. **Journal of Adolescent Health Care.** 1983 Sep;4(3):158-62.

The family planning program of an adolescent care clinic (ACC) was evaluated to determine its effect on the teenage birth rate. The first evaluation compared the teenage birth rate for the target area served by the ACC with a matched area for four years before the ACC began offering services (pre-intervention) and four years after (post-intervention).   The two groups did not differ for the pre-intervention period, but the ACC target area had a lower birth rate for the post-intervention period (p=.015).   The second evaluation was designed to compare the teenage birth rate within the target area for adolescents using the ACC and those not using the service for one year. Adjusting

for   age and race,   the rate for the ACC was 58 per 1,000 births
and for the non-ACC group,   112 per 1,000 births (p<.001).   With
regard   to   ethnic   group differences,   the live birth   rate   for
blacks and Hispanics are very similar.   The adjusted   illegitimate rate for blacks, however, is 76 per 1,000, and the rate for
Hispanics   is 27 per 1,000,   a difference that is significant at
the   p<0.001 level.   This difference is presumably   related   to
different   attitudes in these two cultures toward out-of-wedlock
births.

247.   *Rothenberg PB ;   Philliber SG.   The Young Adult Clinic:
eighteen   months of a contracep-ive and counseling   service   for
young people,   October 1977 to march 1979. New York City, Columbia University,   Center for Population and Family Health.   1979.
41 p.

A Young Adult Clinic designed to give specialized counseling and
contraceptive   services to adolescents was opened at the Presbyterian   Hospital   in 1977.   The clinic program is   designed   to
reduce the incidence of unwanted and unplanned pregnancies among
adolescents   in northern Manhattan.   Visits to the clinic   have
increased by 300% since its first three months of operation.   In
its first 18 months,   there have been 3,652 visits to the clinic
by   1,508   patients,   most of them 16 to 18 years   old,   female,
black   or Hispanic,   living in Manhattan,   not receiving   public
assistance,   and currently enrolled in school.   By their initial
clinic   visit,   44% of all female patients have   been   pregnant.
The   majority   of   these have given birth,   but about   42%   have
resolved their pregnancies by abortion.   Blacks and whites   are
more   likely than Hispanics to be seeking contraception on their
first visit,   while more Hispanics than others come for pregnancy
tests.   Black   patients are most likely to choose   pills   while
Hispanics   are least likely to do so.   Twice the proportion   of
the white patients,   as blacks or Hispanics,   choose diaphragms.
In addition,   white patients are less likely to rely on foam and
condoms than either of the other two groups.

248.   *Schwartz   DB ;   Darabi KF.   Motivations for   adolescents'
first visits to birth control clinics. **Adolescence.** Forthcoming,
1986.

Between   November   1983 and April 1984,   150 young   women   were
interviewed   who   were making their first visits   to   the   Young
Adult Clinic (YAC) at the Presbyterian Hospital in New York City
to   learn   what   motivating factors or events   influenced   their
decisions   to   seek fertility-related services on a   given   day.
The average age at the time of first intercourse for all of   the
young women   in the sample was about 16 years,   although   black
adolescent   contraceptive clients tended to be slightly   younger
than Hispanics (predominantly **Dominicans** and **Puerto Ricans**).   By
the   time they made their first visits to the YAC,   the   average
Hispanic   adolescent was almost 19 and the average black   adolescent was almost 18.   Hispanic teenagers who came to the clinic
for   birth control were much more likely to have   experienced   a
prior   pregnancy than were black teens who came for that reason.
Very   high proportions of teens in both ethnic   groups   reported
having thought that they were pregnant.   Over one-third of each
group   had   been to another birth control clinic   and   over   two-
thirds   had   used a method before coming to   the   YAC.   Roughly
similar proportions of black and Hispanic birth control   clients
said   their parents knew of their clinic visits and low   proportions   of blacks and Hispanic teens had ever worried about   some-

one finding out that they had been to the clinic, about method side effects, or about what would happen during the clinic visit. Clinic related reasons for visits to YAC predominated in both groups. These included recently finding out the clinic existed and the convenience of clinic hours and location.

249. *Torres A ; Forrest JD. Family planning clinic services in the United States: 1983. **Family Planning Perspectives.** 1985 Jan/Feb;17(1):30-5.

Almost five million women were enrolled in family planning clinics in the United States in 1983, eight percent more than in 1981. The number of family planning provider agencies declined slighty, from 2,504 to 2,462, but the number of clinic sites that could be identified increased slightly, from 5,124 to 5,174. About one in 20 women who are exposed to the risk of unintended pregnancy and live in unserved counties are teenagers or low income women. Overall, there are 417,000 low income women and 249,000 teenagers at risk of unintended pregnancy living in counties where there are no family planning clinics. Family planning clinics continue to serve primarily low income women. About 1.6 million women aged 19 and younger were served, representing one-third of all clinic patients in 1983. In 1983, an estimated 532,000 patients (11% of the total) were of Hispanic origin. Hispanic women represented the single highest proportion of all patients served in four of the states along the **Mexican** border: New Mexico (57%), Texas (42%), California (30%), and Arizona (26%). Overall, 44% of all low income women and 31% of teenage women exposed to the risk of unintended pregnancy are served by organized family planning programs.

250. Udry JR. Previous use of medical sources of contraception by newly delivered mothers: 1970. Chapel Hill, North Carolina, University of North Carolina, Family Planning Evaluation Project Report, No. 2-71. April, 1971. 4 p.

During 1970 the author interviewed more than 8,000 mothers in 18 cities in about 60 hospitals and asked them "Before this last pregnancy, did you ever get a birth control method from a public clinic, hospital, private doctor?" The first thing that became evident was that in 1970 very few women were receiving family planning services from hospitals whatever their admission status. For blacks and Spanish mothers, about two women receive public clinic services for every woman receiving private physician contraceptive services. For whites, about three times as many clinic patients received family planning through private physicians as through public clinics. Among white mothers, twice as many private patients as clinic patients had used private physicians for birth control services. Among blacks, three times as many private patients as clinic patients had used private physician contraceptive services, and among Spanish women, five times as many private patients as clinic patients had used private physician services for contraception. Hardly any white private patients had ever used a public clinic for contraception, while a sizable proportion of black and Spanish private patients had used public clinics for this purpose.

251. U.S. Department of Commerce, National Technical Information Services. **Family planning study.** National Analysts, Inc. 1973. 110 p.

This is a study to determine the impact of federally supported

family planning programs in terms of patient satisfaction with
services, utilization of federally assisted family planning projects, program effect on contraceptive behavior, the need for
federal assistance in providing family planning services, and
the reduction of unwanted pregnancies. Relevant chapters discuss sources of family planning services and the demographic
characteristics of clients.   Data include **Mexicans, Puerto
Ricans,** and **Cubans.**

252. *U.S. Department of Health and Human Services, Health
Resources Administration. **Health status of minorities and low
income groups.** By: Rudov MH and Santangelo N. U.S. Government
Printing Office. 1985. 275 p. (Second edition).

Questions of achieving a more equitable access to health care
for all segments of the population are addressed in this report
commissioned by the Office of Health Resources Opportunity in
1977.   Data are presented on the health status of the disadvantaged in reference to vital statistics, reproductive and genetic
health, acute disease conditions, chronic disease conditions,
accidents and injuries, mental health, dental health, preventive
health, utilization of health services, and financial expendi-
tures for health services. For as long as data have been available, non-whites have had higher birth rates than whites. They
have also had a higher share of maternity related and other
reproductive health problems.   Teenage pregnancy and out-of-
wedlock births are two health problems which have increased over
the past decade, and they have negatively affected maternal and
child health among whites, as well as non-whites. With respect
to teenage birth rates, the non-white rate has been approximately twice as high as the white rate, and in the early teens
the differential is even greater.

253. *U.S. Department of Health and Human Services, National
Center for Health Statistics. Basic data on visits to family
planning services sites. By: Hudson BL. **Vital and Health Statistics.** 1982 Jul;13(68):1-32.

Cross-tabulations of data from the National Reporting System for
Family Planning Services are presented.   Information was collected on the sociodemographic characteristics of patients as
well as family planning service utilization.   A sample of private facilities as well as those supported by Public Health
Services family planning grants were selected to participate in
the survey.   The data estimate 9,261,000 family planning visits
were made in 1980, of which only 19% were first visits. Eighty-
nine percent of the visits were made by women under the age of
30; teenagers comprised one-third of this group.   Women of
Hispanic origin made 13% of the total visits.   Ninety percent of
the visits made by Hispanics were made by women with 12 years of
education or less, and 13% of the Hispanic clients were from
families receiving public assistance.   Fifty-eight percent of
the white women, 44% of the black women, and 23% of the Hispanic
women were nulliparous.   In 84% of their visits some method of
contraception was adopted or continued by Hispanic women (60%
chose the pill, 13% the IUD, and three percent diaphragms).
Prior contraceptive method was reported by 82% of the whites,
83% of the blacks, and 81% of the Hispanics.

254. *U.S. Department of Health and Human Services, National
Center for Health Statistics. Basic data on women who use family
planning clinics: United States, 1980. By: Bloom B. **Vital and**

Health Statistics. 1982;13(67). 46 p.

This report presents basic data on women who used organized family planning clinics in the United States during 1980. The statistics based on data collected from the National Reporting System for Family Planning Services focus on the socioeconomic characteristics, pregnancy history, and contraceptive methods of women patients. The report includes the following tables by number of female family planning patients: age; patient status; ethnicity; education; race; public assistance status; prior contraceptive use; medical services provided; and number of pregnancies, live births, and abortions. Separate findings are reported for Hispanic clients.

255. *U.S. Department of Health and Human Services, National Center for Health Statistics. Family planning visits by teenagers: United States, 1978. By: Foster J and Eckard E. **Vital and Health Statistics.** 1981 Aug;13(58):1-24.

Data from the 1978 National Reporting System for Family Planning Services are reported. The bulk of the family planning visits (56%) were concentrated among teenagers 18 or 19 years old. About nine percent of the visits were made by patients under age 16. The proportion of visits by white teenagers was 68% compared with 31% by black teenagers. However, the visit rate per 1,000 population was much higher for black than for white teenagers. About six percent of the visits were made by teenagers of Hispanic origin or descent. Sixty-two percent of the visits were made by those who had not yet completed high school. Visits made by members of families receiving public assistance income were about as common among teenagers (15%) as among women of all ages (15%). Sixty-four percent of the visits were made by teenagers who had never been pregnant. Twenty-eight percent of all visits and 65% of initial visits were associated with teenagers who had never regularly used a contraceptive method. Sixty percent of all visits were made by teenagers who reported the oral contraceptive as their prior method. Adoption or continuation of the oral contraceptive occurred at 77% of the teenagers' family planning visits. Adoption or continuation of the IUD, diaphragm, and foam/jelly/cream each accounted for about four percent of all teenagers' visits.

256. U.S. Department of Health and Human Services, National Center for Health Statistics. **National Reporting System for Family Planning Services: 1974 annual report.** U.S. DHEW. May, 1977. 245 p.; and ---, **National Reporting System for Family Planning Services: 1975 annual report.** U.S. DHEW. September, 1977. 245 p.

The National Center for Health Statistics (NCHS) has been operating a reporting system for family planning services since May 1969. Most family planning service sites that receive federal funds for service report to NCHS. The Clinic Visit Record for Family Planning Services is the basic collection form and includes social, demographic, and family planning service information. The tables presented in the reports are produced from data collected during the given year. The numbers and characteristics of the patients who received family planning services during the year are shown for both the United States as a whole and for each individual state. Separate data for Latin Americans are included.

257.   *U.S.   Department of Health and Human   Services,   National
Center for Health Statistics.   Patient profile, National Report-
ing System for Family Planning Services: United States,   1978.
By: Foster JE. **Advance Data.** 1981 Jun;73. 7 p.

The National Reporting System for Family Planning Services began
in 1972 to collect data on clinic based visits for family planning services in the United States and some of its territories,
and encompasses family planning visits occurring in clinics.
Data collected for the year 1978 are presented in this report.
Information on the numbers of patients, patient status, female
patient demographics, pregnancy history, and contraceptive use
is given.   Although there are proportionately more white than
black female patients (69% and 29% respectively), the black
enrollment rate is 181 per 1,000 women aged 15 to 44 years
compared with the white enrollment rate of 61 per 1,000 women
aged 15 to 44 years.   Women of Hispanic origin comprise 11% of
all female patients, with an enrollment rate of 133 per 1,000
women aged 15 to 44 years.   There are at least two times as many
white as black female patients in the youngest age group.   A
smaller proportion of teenage women in the youngest age group
was reported as being of Hispanic origin or descent than were
women in the two older age groups.

258.   *U.S.   Department of Health and Human Services,   National
Center for Health Statistics.   Patterns of ambulatory care in
obstetrics and gynecology: the National Ambulatory Medical Care
Survey.   By: Cypress B. **Vital and Health Statistics.** 1984
Feb;13(76).

Data on the ambulatory medical care provided during office
visits to obstetrician/gynecologists are presented.   Individual
practice profiles are drawn for different age groups of physicians, for those in the four major geographic regions, for those
in metropolitan and non-metropolitan areas, and for those in
solo and group practices.   Patterns of medical care are also
described according to the age of the patient and prior visit
status.   Descriptors of practice include patients' reasons for
visit and diagnoses rendered by physicians.   Data on the utilization of patient management techniques include diagnostic services, medication therapy, and non-medication therapy.   In the
National Ambulatory Medical Care Survey about six percent of all
female visits to obstetrician/gynecologists were made by Hispanic patients, compared with five percent of female visits to
all specialists, a small but statistically significant difference.   Black females visited obstetrician/ gynecologists in
about the same proportion as they visited all specialists.
Although general visit rates did not vary significantly by race
or ethnicity, black females 15 to 24 years of age visited at a
lower rate than white females, and Hispanic females 25 to 44
years of age visited at a lower rate than non-Hispanic females.

259.   *U.S.   Department of Health and Human Services, National
Center for Health Statistics. **Provisional data from the National
Reporting System for Family Planning Services: January 1973 to
December 1973, United States, states, and territories.** Washing-
ton D.C. 1974. 350 p.

Data are tabulated from 4,067 clinics in the fifty United
States, the District of Columbia, Puerto Rico, Guam, and the
Virgin Islands, covering 2,138,410 patients who made almost
3,500,000 visits, primarily for female contraceptive services.

Tables include data on race, Latin American origin (including **Mexicans** and **Puerto Ricans**), number of patients, types of services, fertility, past and current contraceptive use and method changes, and background characteristics. Both national level and state level data are presented.

260. *U.S. Department of Health and Human Services, National Center for Health Statistics. Use of family planning services by currently married women 15 to 44 years of age: United States, 1973 and 1976. By: Hendershot GE. **Advance Data.** 1979 Feb;45:1-10.

The National Survey of Family Growth conducted by the National Center for Health Statistics was designed to provide data on fertility, family planning and related aspects of maternal and child health. In 1976, 59% of white women, 51% of Hispanic women and 46% of black women reported family planning visits. In all groups the last family planning visit was more likely to be with their own physician as opposed to organized medical services, though the latter had a larger share of last visits among black women (37%), and Hispanic women (33%) compared to white women (14%). Women aged 15 to 24 are more likely to report a family planning visit and women 35 to 44 were least likely. This is true in both surveys and among most ethnic and income groups. In both age groups, 25 to 34, and 35 to 44, about one in eight last visits were to an organized medical service in 1976, about the same as in 1973. For the age group 15 to 24, the visits to organized medical services were about one in five. The proportion of teenage wives reporting a family planning visit in the three year period before the interview increased from 70% to 77% between 1973 and 1976.

261. *U.S. Department of Health and Human Services, National Center for Health Statistics. Use of services for family planning and infertility: United States. By: Hendershot GE and Bauman KE. **Vital and Health Statistics.** 1981 Dec;23(8):1-15.

The statistics presented in this report on the use of family planning and infertility services in the United States are based on interviews with a national sample of 6,428 currently married women 15 to 44 years of age, which were conducted by the National Center for Health Statistics. Most non-sterile married women had talked with a physician or other professional about family planning in the three years before their interview in 1976 (59%). Recent family planning visits were more common among white women (60%), than among black (47%), or Hispanic women (52%). Younger women (15 to 29 years of age) were more likely than older women (30 to 44 years of age) to have made a recent family planning visit (71% and 45%, respectively). This difference by age existed independently of race or ethnicity. Recent visitors who were black or Hispanic women, were more likely than white recent visitors to have made their latest visit to an organized medical service. Young visitors were more likely to have gone to organized medical services (18%) than older women (12%).

262. *U.S. Department of Health and Human Services, National Center for Health Statistics. Use of services for family planning and infertility: United States, 1982. By: Horn MC and Mosher WD. **Advance Data from Vital and Health Statistics.** 1984 Dec;103. 8 p.

The 1982 statistics on the use of family planning and infertility services presented in this report are preliminary results
from Cycle III of the National Survey of Family Growth conducted
by the National Center for Health Statistics.   Overall,   79% of
currently married non-sterile women reported using some type   of
family planning service during the previous three years.   There
were   no   statistically   significant differences   between   white
(79%),   black (75%) or Hispanic (77%) wives,   or between the two
income   groups.   The annual rate of visits for family   planning
services   in 1982 was 1,077 visits per 1,000 women.   Teenagers
had   the highest annual visit rate (1,581 per 1,000) of any   age
group   for   all sources of family planning services combined.
Visit   rates declined sharply with age from 1,447 at ages 15   to
24,   to 479 at ages 35 to 44.   Data were also collected in 1982
on   use   of   medical services for infertility by women   who   had
difficulty in conceiving or carrying a pregnancy to term.   About
one   million   ever   married women had one   or   more   infertility
visits in the 12 months before the interview.   During the three
years before the interview,   about 1.9 million women had   infertility visits.

263.   *U.S.   Department   of Health and Human Services,   National
Center· for Health Statistics.   Utilization of   family   planning
services   by   currently   married women 15 to 44   years   of   age:
United States,   1973. By: Notzon F. **Vital and Health Statistics.**
1977 Nov;23(1). 36p.

This study is based on data collected in Cycle I of the National
Survey   of   Family Growth,   a periodic survey conducted   by   the
National   Center for Health Statistics.   The following were included among the survey findings: 1) 54% of currently   married
women   aged   15 to 44 talked at least once with a   physician   or
other   trained person about family planning methods in the   five
years   preceding   the 1973 interview;   2) for currently   married
women over the age of 20,   the percentage with a family planning
visit   in the last five years declined significantly   with   each
successive   older age group;   3) there was a significant difference between the percentage of white women and black women   with
a   visit in the last five years (55% for white women and 46% for
black women);   4) among women of Spanish origin,   51% reported at
least one family planning visit in the last five years;   5)   the
percentage   of both white and black women with a family planning
visit   in   the last five years did not vary   significantly   with
total   family   income;   6) the proportion of   currently   married
women   with a family planning visit declined with   increases   in
parity;   and   7)   there was not a significant difference in   the
percent   of women with a family planning visit between   Catholic
and Protestant women.

264.   *U.S.   Department   of Health and Human Services,   National
Center·for Health Statistics. Visits to family planning clinics:
United States,   1979. By: Bloom B. **Advance Data.** 1981 Sep;74(4):
1-8.

The   National Reporting System for Family Planning   Services   is
conducted   by   the   Division of Health Care   Statistics   of   the
United States National Center for Health Statistics.   Since mid-
1977,   the system has been conducted as a sample survey,   involving   a   sampling   of clinics and a sampling of   clients   at   the
chosen   clinics.   This   is a report of visits made by women   to
family   planning   clinics   in the U.S. in 1979.   Women   made
8,609,000   visits   to family planning clinics in 1979,   a   16%

increase over the number of visits in 1978.   This increase was largely due to the addition of 169 service sites during the year.   Eighty-nine percent of all visits were made by women under 30.   Seventy percent were made by white women and 12% by Hispanic women.   Women living on public assistance income accounted for 14% of all visits to family planning clinics, the percentage increasing with the age of the woman.   Forty-three percent of all visits were made by women who had never been pregnant.   During 93% of the visits, a method of contraception was adopted or continued.   Oral contraceptives were the overwhelming choice of women (68%) of all classes, ages, races, and ethnic backgrounds. This was particularly true for teenagers.

265. *U.S. Department of Health and Human Services, National Center· for Health Statistics. Women who use organized family planning services: United States, 1979. By: Eckard E. **Vital and Health Statistics.** 1982;13(62). 27 p.

A descriptive analysis is made of women who visited organized family planning clinics in 1979.   The social and demographic characteristics of the women are related to their pregnancy and contraceptive histories and to the types of services received during their visits.   Statistics are based on data from the National Reporting System for Family Planning Services and other data sources from the National Center for Health Statistics. Close to 12% of the family planning patients were of Hispanic origin, with an enrollment of 143 per 1,000 women 15 to 44 years of age.   The pill was the method adopted by 64% of the women and was the method most often adopted by women in all age groups. Women of Hispanic origin differ significantly from other women in the proportion of women who have had at least one pregnancy and at least one live birth.   About half of the Hispanic women under 20 have had at least one pregnancy.

266. Urdaneta ML. Fertility regulation among Mexican American women in an urban setting: a comparison of indigent versus non-indigent Chicanos in a southwest city in the United States. Doctoral Dissertation, Southern Methodist University. 1976. 281 p. DAI;38(3-A):1507).

The effect of a recently instituted federally subsidized family planning clinic on the fertility of medically indigent Chicanos in a southwestern city was examined and the data were compared with that obtained from Chicano college graduates and members of a local **Mexican** American Business and Professional Women's Association.   The indigent Chicano woman was eager to regulate fertility, particularly when the regimen was sensitively presented, inexpensive, and placed in the context of a total family health program.   College graduate Chicanos averaged one child per woman, a figure lower than that of the general American population.   It is contended that cultural arguments explaining the exceptionally high fertility rate of Mexican Americans are not valid for this population, and that Roman Catholicism was not a deterrent to family planning, nor is the concept of machismo.   The problem instead appears to stem from the disjuncture of the Anglo system of implementing family planning services with this ethnic group and the Mexican American'.s perception of service utilization.

2. Contraceptive Use: Reversible Methods

267. *Andrade SJ. Contraceptive use by adolescents: what do we know about Chicanas? Paper presented at the Annual Meeting of the American Educational Research Association, Los Angeles, California. (Unpublished) April, 1981. 33 p.

The primary objective of this field work in a family planning clinic was to assess the quality of contraceptive education and clinic services available to adolescents in a Texan community of about 346,000 inhabitants, and to survey what teenagers themselves viewed as barriers to information about reproduction, contraception, and contraceptive services. Results indicate that the young Chicanas appeared highly motivated in terms of their return to the birth control clinic; the majority with their parents' knowledge and many with their families' active support. Over 80% agreed that the best time to start childrearing would be between the ages of 19 and 24, most wanting only two children. The impressions of health care providers fell into two main distinct groups. The larger group tended to describe **Mexican** American teens largely in terms of familial or cultural explanations, attributing difficulties of young women to the influence of their families or to some norms or values of the Mexican American culture. The small group of Mexican American health providers believed that young Mexican American females continue to have very few social and economic options available to them beyond the role of motherhood.

268. Andrade SJ ; Jones V. Family planning attitudes and practices as a function of the degree of cultural identification of female Mexican American college students. Doctoral Dissertation, Austin, Texas, University of Texas. 1979. 240 p. DAI;40(3-B):1418.

The extent to which identification with traditional **Mexican** American culture affects the attitudes of female Mexican American college students toward family planning and contraceptives was investigated. Subjects were 150 female Mexican American students at two Texas universities. Data also include **Puerto Rican** women. A causal model was postulated that a woman's

cultural identity would condition her attitudes toward family
planning which in turn would influence her use of contraceptives.   The results did not support this model, and an alternative was developed,   incorporating significant attitudinal and
exogenous variables to explain the women's use of contraceptives.   The single strongest predictor of contraceptive use was
whether or not the woman was having regular sexual relations.
This variable was unrelated to cultural identification.   Concerns about population as a social and economic issue were the
major attitudinal factors influencing women's use of contraception.

269. Bennett CF. Lateness of contraception among recipients of
subsidized family planning services. **American Journal of Public
Health.** 1970 Nov;60(11):2110-17.

At the Planned Parenthood Center in Tucson, Arizona, a 1967
study was made of files of 507 acceptor/patients, divided in
three cohorts by age, analyzed lateness of contraceptive initiation with respect to race/ethnicity, years of formal education,
birth cohort, and source of referral to the Center.   It is
estimated that 30% did not begin contraception until after
having five or more children, and 18% did not until after six or
more.   Anglos began contraception earliest, followed by **Mexican**
Americans, with blacks last. Low education seems to account for
late contraception among all Mexican American patients and among
most younger black patients.   From 1962 to 1967, two sources of
referral related to lateness of contraception were Planned Parenthood Center publicity (patients less likely to have five or
more children at contraceptive initiation) and health or welfare
agencies (referred patients more likely to have five or more
children at first use).   Educational level and racial/ethnic
identity were also related to source of referral.   Late initiation of contraception could possibly be prevented through expansion of subsidized family planning services with programs
encouraging high school completion.

270. *Cummings M ; Cummings S. Family planning among the urban
poor: sexual politics and social policy. **Family Relations.** 1983
Jan;31(1):47-58.

This paper examines several of the myths and stereotypes associated with the sexual and reproductive behavior of the urban
poor.   Particular attention is given to the birth control and
reproductive practices of poor white, black, and **Mexican** American women.   Some values that are supposedly prominent in the
Mexican American culture are strongly tied to traditional sex
roles.   For example, a recent study of Mexican American families in Austin, Texas, concluded that barriers of communication
between husbands and wives seemed particularly strong in the
areas of family size and sexual behavior.   The husband's attitude toward birth control appeared to be a crucial factor in
determining female access to family planning services.   While
the machismo ethic may be more applicable to Mexican American
culture, it is difficult to conclude with certainty that chau-
vinism is any weaker in the black and white male population.
Children apparently occupy a central place in the Mexican American family, and are a source of satisfaction for the mother.
Based on cultural and historical traditions, some scholars suggest that for many Mexican American women bearing children is a
very important source of fulfillment.

271. *Ezzati I ;   Russell Briefel R ;   Perlman J. Selected contraceptive and health practices of Mexican American women: Hispanic Health and Nutrition Examination Survey,   southwest United
States, 1982-1984. Paper presented at the 113th Annual Meeting
of the American Public Health Association,   Washington, D.C. November 17-21, 1985.

Prevalence rates of various contraceptive methods for **Mexican**
American females aged 12 to 74 years were estimated using data
from the first phase of the Hispanic Health and   Nutrition
Examination Survey (HHANES:1982-84).   The prevalence of oral
contraceptive use among premenopausal Mexican American women
aged 15 to 44 years was 19% overall, and highest in the age
groups 20 to 29 years (28%), and 30 to 34 years (22%).   Compared
to oral contraceptive use data for whites and blacks from HHANES
II (1976-80), Mexican American women have a similar pattern of
pill use.   Tubal ligation, another popular method of birth
control in the general population (12% in women aged 15 to 44
years in 1982) was found in 15% of Mexican American women aged
15 to 44 years.   For adult women aged 20 to 74 years, recommended screening intervals were not met by 23% and 27% for a Pap
smear and a breast examination, respectively.   The association
between these contraceptive and health practices will be discussed in relationship to the utilization of health services and
with respect to socioeconomic characteristics such as income,
education, and acculturation.

272. *Fielder EP ; Becerra RM. Contraceptive use among Mexican
American adolescent females. Paper presented at the 113th Annual
Meeting of the American Public Health Association, Washington,
D.C. November 17-21, 1985.

It appears that the increasing levels of sexual activity among
adolescent never married women have been accompanied by an
increasing use of contraception.   The trend in contraceptive
use, however, while difficult to document, has primarily been
studied with black and/or white populations.   Very little is
known about contraceptive use among Hispanic adolescents.   The
specific aim of this paper is to examine similarities and differences in contraceptive use among **Mexican** Americans compared
to Anglo Americans.   Issues identified and discussed are the
role of peers, familial attitudes, and the individual's own
knowledge base.   These issues are analyzed with respect to
varying levels of acculturation and socioeconomic status.   The
data are based on a community survey of 1,000 adolescent females, aged 13 to 19 (700 Mexican Americans and 300 Anglo Americans).   The sample was selected through multi-stage probability
sampling techniques using 1980 Los Angeles County Census data.

273. *Gibbs CE ;   Martin HW ;   Gutierrez M.   Prisoners of hope:
family planning. In: Lewit S, ed. **Advances in planned parenthood, Vol. 8.** Amsterdam, Excerpta Medica. 1973. p. 21-24.

Family planning attitudes and practices among medically indigent
women, particularly **Mexican** Americans, in San Antonio, Texas, is
examined. The study is based on interviews with 381 recently delivered patients at the Robert B. Green Hospital. Seventy-eight
percent were Mexican American.   Ninety-nine percent were under
35 years of age, yet 24% had already given birth to five or more
children and 44% had two to four children.   Forty-two percent
reported that they or their partners had used contraceptives at
some point and 33% were using them in the cycle during which

they conceived.   Of the 58% who had never used contraceptives,
fear and ignorance were among the principal reasons.   Sixty-nine
percent reported they wanted no more children and only six women
said they wanted as many children as they could have.   At the
time of the interview, 93% said they would like to use some form
of contraception, 55% preferring orals, 15% sterilization, and
nearly 15% IUDs.   The women generally seemed well disposed
toward family planning if services could be made available to
them.   On the basis of the study, the authors recommend guidelines for a service project.

274.   *Harvey SM. Trends in contraceptive use at one university:
1974-1978. **Family Planning Perspectives.** 1980 Nov/Dec;12(6):301-
4.

In a group of 2,700 women making initial visits to the contraception clinic at the California State University at Fullerton
between 1974 and 1978, oral contraceptives were the most frequently chosen methods of three prescriptions (the others were
the IUD and diaphragm.)   The proportion of women using the pill,
however, declined sharply over the period, from 89% to 63% of
patients.   Choice of the diaphragm rose substantially, from six
percent to 33%.   The proportion of women choosing the IUD fluc-
tuated over the period, showing no clear trend and averaging
eight percent.   The decline in the proportion of women choosing
the pill was sharpest among white Anglo students (down from 85%
to 63%).   Among non-whites and Hispanics, the proportion fell
from 89% to 80%.   The increase in the choice of the diaphragm
was also greatest among the Anglo students.   These trends of decreased choice of the pill and increased acceptance of the
diaphragm are much sharper than those shown among young married
women at the national level.

275.   *Holck SE ; Rochat RW ; Warren CW ; Friedman J ; Smith JC.
Use of reproductive health services along the United States/
Mexican border: results of a household probability survey. Pre-
sented at the 108th Annual Meeting of the American Public Health
Association, Detroit, Michigan.   (Unpublished) October 19-23,
1980. 3 p.

In 1979 the Centers for Disease Control conducted a maternal and
child health and family planning survey among a sample of 2,135
women living in the United States/**Mexican** border states of
Texas, New Mexico, Arizona, and California.   Of the 2,135 women,
37% were Anglo, 59% were Hispanic, and four percent were black.
Major findings were: 1) the Hispanics had experienced an average of 4.8 births and the Anglos had experienced an average of
3.1 births; 2) 53% of the Hispanics and 43% of the Anglos indicated their last pregnancy was unplanned; 3) 60% of all Anglo
women and 46% of all Hispanic women were currently practicing
contraception; 4) among currently married women only, 75% of the
Anglos and 66% of the Hispanics were currently practicing contraception; 5) among never married women, 26% of the Anglos and
13% of the Hispanics were currently practicing contraception; 6)
sterilization and oral contraceptives were the most popular
contraceptive methods among both groups, but male sterilization
was more common among the Anglos than among the Hispanics; 7)
nine percent of the currently married Hispanics and five percent
of the previously married Hispanics obtained their contraceptives by crossing the border into Mexico, while the remainder of
the Hispanics and all of the Anglos obtained their contraceptives in the U.S.

276.   *Holck SE ;   Warren CW ;   Morris L ;   Rochat RW.   Need for
family   planning   services   among Anglo and   Hispanic   women   in
United   States counties bordering Mexico. **Family Planning Perspectives.** 1982 May/Jun;14(3):155-9.

Although family planning services have been available in the
United States/Mexico border area for more than a decade, some
groups of women are still in need of services.   A survey of
women of reproductive age living on the U.S. side of the U.S./
Mexico border indicates that 19% of ever married Hispanic women
and eight percent of Anglos at risk of unintended pregnancy were
not using contraceptives.   Among Hispanics, levels of unmet need
were highest among women aged 35 to 44, those with four or more
children and those with fewer than eight years of education;
among Anglos,   unmet need was highest among women aged 15 to 34,
those with two or fewer children and those with less than a high
school education.   Hispanics were much more likely than Anglos
to patronize organized family planning programs (34% vs. six
percent).

277.   *Lindemann C ;   Scott W. The fertility-related behavior of
Mexican American adolescents. **Journal of Early Adolescence.**
1982;2(1):31-8.

Data from a clinic sample of pregnant adolescents are analyzed
for differences in fertility-related variables between **Mexican**
Americans and non-Mexicans.   The independent variables are birth
place, ethnicity, and exposure to United States culture of Mexican and non-Mexican adolescents.   The dependent variables are
talking about sex, pregnancy, birth control, hearing about birth
control, and use of birth control.   The data support the hypothesis that in the process of acculturation the fertility-
related behavior of immigrant Mexican adolescent females is
affected by the indigenous U.S./Mexican culture rather than by
U.S. Anglo culture.   Implications for delivery of services are
discussed.   The delivery of fertility related services should
take into account the cultural preferences of Mexican women, and
should not involve coercion from legal or medical authorities.
While liberation of Mexican American women, and accompanying
changes in childbearing patterns may be desirable, these efforts
should originate within the Mexican American community.   Data
are presented in tables on selected sample and subsample characteristics and compares fertility behaviors across ethnic groups,
including Anglo, black, U.S. non-Mexican, and U.S. Mexican.

278.   Linn MW ;   Gurel L ;   Carmichael JS ;   Klitenick P ;   Shane R.
Cross-cultural comparison of birth control effectiveness.   Paper
presented at the 104th Annual Meeting of the American Public
Health Association, Miami Beach, Florida. October 17-21, 1976.
14 p.

A total of 449 mothers, aged 35 to 45, from four subcultural
groups and the white, Protestant majority cultural group were
studied in the Miami, Florida area to determine the relationship
of attitudes to contraceptive behavior.   The women were randomly
selected from black, **Cuban,** Indian (Miccosukee and Seminole),
and migrant Chicano (**Mexican**) populations. About one-third used
very effective birth control practices and 28% used no method at
all.   The white group was the only group that almost always used
some method of contraception.   The Cubans were the only group
almost never using pills or IUDs.   The greatest predictor of
effective contraception was use of birth control before first

pregnancy (p<.01).   Cubans were the most negative of all groups
toward abortion, but were the only group reporting abortion to
any extent; Chicanos and Cubans were most negative toward birth
control, and also were the most likely to be Catholic.   Negative
attitudes predicted using no method at all except in the Chicanos; also, high negative attitudes were found among Cubans who
used the pill and IUD.   In most of the subcultures the mothers
wanted large numbers of children, knew of effective methods of
birth control, and chose not to use them.

279. Mosher WD ; Bacharach CA. First premarital contraceptive
use in the United States: determinants and trends, 1960s-1982.
Paper presented at the Annual Meeting of the Population Association of America. April, 1986.

Teenage pregnancy rates in the United States exceed those of
other Western industrialized countries, probably because of low
levels of contraceptive use among women having premarital sex
(Jones et al., 1985). This study shows the first national estimates of trends and differentials in first use of contraception
for a national sample of all women.   Data are from the National
Survey of Family Growth, Cycle III, 1982.   The percentage of
women who used (or whose partners used) contraception at first
premarital sex increased from the early 1960s to the late 1970s,
but only because of an increase in use of withdrawal.   However,
in the early 1980s, use at first intercourse increased sharply
because of an increase in use of the condom. The proportion who
used a method at first sex varied from 23% among Hispanic women,
to 74% among Jewish women; it was higher among white than black
women, and higher in higher socioeconomic categories.   After
first intercourse, contraceptive use did not vary significantly
by socioeconomic characteristics.   While the condom and withdrawal were leading methods at first intercourse, women who used
their first method after their first intercourse overwhelmingly
chose the pill.

280. Nies CM. Social psychological variables related to family
planning among Mexican American females. Doctoral Dissertation,
Austin, Texas, University of Texas. (Unpublished) 1974. No. 74-
24,914.

Social psychological variables related to family planning were
investigated in **Mexican** American females contacted immediately
following delivery at a Texas county hospital.   The dependent
variable was use of either the birth control pill or intrauter-
ine device two months following delivery.   Wife's perception of
husband's feelings was the strongest single predictor of later
contraceptive practice, suggesting the need for including husbands in birth planning programs. Within marital status, single
women had a much lower success rate than married women, apparently due to the intentions not to have additional intercourse
prior to marriage.   Intentions to use specific methods were
moderately related to later use of those methods.   The more
modern women, as measured by the personal values abstract,
tended to adopt birth planning methods with greater frequency,
and a dichotomized version of the pill had a superior correlation on cross validation.

281. *Philliber SG ; Namerow PB ; Kaye JW ; Kunkes CH. Pregnancy risk taking among adolescents. Paper presented at the 1984
Annual Meeting of the Population Association of America, Minneapolis, Minnesota. May 3-5, 1984. 9 p.

This research tests the utility of Kristin Luker's cost benefit theory which posits that at each coital event a cost benefit set toward contraceptive use and pregnancy is operative. Luker suggests that when the perceived probability of pregnancy is low and the probability assigned to abortion is high, risk taking is more likely. The data come from interviews with 425 teenage women in New York. The findings offer support for the Luker model, since in an equation also including background variables and level of ego development, four of six Luker variables (the subjective probabilities of pregnancy and abortion, and the disadvantages of pregnancy and birth control) were significantly related to pregnancy risk taking. The most parsimonious model to explain risk taking includes five Luker variables, as well as welfare history, a measure of previous risk taking, and level of ego development. In the ethnic comparisons, Hispanic teenagers were more likely than blacks or whites to have risked pregnancy at last coitus.

282. Polgar S ; Rothstein F. Research report: family planning and conjugal roles in New York City poverty areas. **Social Science and Medicine.** 1970 Jul;4:135-9.

The compatibility between methods of birth control and conjugal role relationships was investigated in New York City in a research project initiated in 1965 by the Planned Parenthood Federation of America. Among both blacks and **Puerto Ricans,** women reporting a joint relationship had fewer children, with age controlled, than those with separated female-dominant conjugal roles. Natality was higher among Puerto Rican women reporting male-dominant rather than female-dominant separated relationships. Among blacks, those in separated roles were more likely than those in joint roles to be using the coitus independent methods in 1965 and to have switched to them more often. Among Puerto Ricans, all three conjugal role groups had switched from coitus connected female methods, but the women reporting joint relationships were more likely to be using the pill or IUD than those with separated roles.

283. *Pomeroy R ; Torres A. Family planning practices of low income women in two communities. **American Journal of Public Health.** 1972;62:1123-9.

A sample of 1,351 white, black and Spanish American women between the ages of 18 and 44 from the low income districts of Grand Rapids, Michigan and Albuquerque, New Mexico were interviewed regarding their use of contraception. Findings indicate that except for white women in Albuquerque, about one-third of the sample had never used contraception. The majority of each subsample were either now using or had used contraception in the past. Black and Spanish American women were less likely to be or to have been users of contraception than their white counterparts and were more likely to be at risk of an unwanted pregnancy. The poor generally used contraception as much or more than the women of low marginal incomes. Of all women using contraception at the time of the interview, over half were using oral contraception. Despite family planning clinics in the area, two-thirds of the poor white subsamples and two-thirds of the users of contraception received their first prescription from a private doctor. For all ethnic subsamples, the low marginal income respondents used public medical sources less than the poor.

284. *Pratt WF ; Mosher WD ; Bacharach CA ; Horn MC. Under-
standing United States fertility: findings from the National
Survey of Family Growth, Cycle III. **Population Bulletin.** 1984
Dec;39(5):3-42.

The first overview of findings from Cycle III of the National
Survey of Family Growth, the latest of seven such surveys of
United States fertility since 1955 and the first to cover all
women of childbearing age in the coterminous U.S. is presented.
Interviews between August 1982 and February 1983 with 7,969
women, representative of 54 million women aged 15 to 44, reveal
that sterilization is now the leading contraceptive method in
the U.S. (22%, female sterilization; 11% male sterilization),
followed by the pill (29%), condom (12%), diaphragm (eight
percent), and IUD (seven percent). Only 45% of women aged 15 to
44 in 1982 had used a contraceptive method at first intercourse.
Four out of five women married for the first time between 1975
and 1982 had intercourse before marriage. Hispanic women are
more likely than non-Hispanic women to have had a first child
before marriage (28% compared to 17%). Approximately one quarter of Hispanic women (25%) aged 15 to 44 used a contraceptive
method at first intercourse compared to 46% of non-Hispanic
women.   Hispanic women made 1,212 family planning visits per
1,000 women who had ever had intercourse, and were not sterile
before February 1979 in the 12 months before the 1982 interview
compared to 1,065 visits per 1,000 women who were non-Hispanic.

285. *Rochat RW ; Warren CW ; Smith JC ; Holck SE ; Friedman
JS. Family planning practices among Anglo and Hispanic women in
United States counties bordering Mexico. **Family Planning Per-
spectives.** 1981 Jul/Aug;13(4):176-80.

The United States Centers for Disease Control surveyed women of
reproductive age living on the U.S. side of the Mexican border
as to contraceptive use and source of care.   It found that
overall contraceptive practice is quite similar among married
Hispanic (**Mexican**) and Anglo (white, non-Hispanic) women; 75% of
Anglo and 66% of Hispanics use some method. Among never mar-
rieds however, Anglos are twice as likely as Hispanics to use a
method.   About 22% of Anglo and 12% of Hispanic women are pro-
tected from pregnancy by contraceptive sterilization of themselves or partners, the difference almost entirely attributable
to a very low incidence of vasectomy among Hispanic males.   The
pill is the most popular reversible method among both groups.
Hispanic women are more likely to go to Planned Parenthood or
health department clinics, and Anglo women are more likely to go
to private physicians or clinics. Unmet need is much higher
among Hispanics; about four times the proportion of married
Hispanic women as comparable Anglo women were at risk of unintended pregnancy and were using no method.

286. *Sabagh G. Fertility planning status of Chicano couples in
Los Angeles. **American Journal of Public Health.** 1980;70(1):56-
61.

Data obtained in interviews of 1,129 Chicanas in an area probability sample of Los Angeles households in 1973 were used to
present estimates of fertility planning status of Chicano (**Mexican**) couples and to identify those dimensions that appear to be
related to the number of planned pregnancies.   The level of
contraceptive use prior to the last pregnancy was found to be
somewhat lower for Chicanas than for all women in the United

States, but they were equally successful in their fertility planning. The success rate for Chicana contraceptors ranged from 65% before the first pregnancy to 42% before the fourth, a little higher than for all women in the U.S. For noncontraceptors, there were similar differences in success between the two groups. The findings suggest that the higher fertility of Chicanas is a consequence of their desire for larger families rather than unsuccessful family planning. Findings on the determinants of fertility planning success suggest that ethnicity and type of health facility care for the last pregnancy are more important variables than age, age at marriage, socioeconomic status, and religiosity.

287. Scott CS. The relationship between beliefs about the menstrual cycle and choice of fertility regulating methods within five ethnic groups. **International Journal of Gynecology and Obstetrics.** 1975;13(3):105-9.

The hypothesis that a woman's concept about her body functions may initiate rejection of certain Fertility Regulating Methods (FRM), specifically of oral contraceptives and IUDs, which modify bodily functions, motivated an investigation among five ethnic populations (Bahamians, **Cubans, Haitians, Puerto Ricans** and South American blacks). The most pronounced theme among the groups was dissatisfaction with those methods which modify menstruation. Ethnically patterned responses showed that an important relationship existed between rejection of those FRMs which modify menstrual bleeding and the various concepts of blood. Irregularity of menstrual processes was viewed among all groups as a threat to health and well being. This investigation suggests that women's concepts of bodily functions are among the major factors influencing their decisions concerning choice, use or non-use of orthodox Fertility Regulating Methods.

288. *Smith JC ; Warren CW ; Garcia Nunez J. The United States/Mexico border: contraceptive use and maternal health care in perspective. El Paso, Texas, United States/Mexico Border Health Association, No. iv. 1983. 110 p.

A household probability survey was conducted from June to September 1979 of 5,005 households in 51 selected counties in the four United States border states of Texas, New Mexico, Arizona, and California. General criteria for inclusion of a county in the survey were proximity to the U.S./Mexico border, and a Spanish surnamed head of household in at least 25% of the households in the county according to the 1970 Census. **Mexican** Americans in the four border states have the highest fertility of any race or ethnic group in the U.S., with a cumulative fertility rate of 4.3 compared with 2.8 for the Anglos in that area, and this is associated with low socioeconomic status. An unwanted most recent live birth was more common among Mexican Americans than among Anglos. Contraceptive use in the border area was high for both ethnic groups and increased with parity, but the percentages for use after the birth of the first child were higher for Anglos than for Mexican Americans. For currently married Mexican Americans, oral contraceptives were the most commonly used contraceptives, followed by sterilization; for Anglos, the reverse was true.

289. *Smith JC ; Warren CW ; Garcia Nunez J ; Rochat RW. Family planning along the United States/Mexico border. Presented at the 109th Annual Meeting of the American Public Health Association,

Los Angeles, California. (Unpublished) November 3, 1981. 13 p.

Tables are presented on family planning along the United States/Mexico border. Sixty-six percent of 804 **Mexican** Americans and 75% of Anglos were currently using contraception. Twenty-four percent of the Mexican Americans and 23% of the Anglos had previously used contraception. Eleven percent of the Mexican Americans and two percent of the Anglos had never used contraception. The percentage distribution of respondents 15 to 44 years of age by contraceptive method, marital status and geographic area is presented. The totals for the border and national samples are as follows: the border - sterilization (22%), injections (six percent), oral contraceptives (40%), IUD (14%), condom (three percent), and other (14%); and the national sample - sterilization (24%), injections (seven percent), oral contraceptives (33%), IUD (16%), condom (two percent), and other (18%). The percent of never married Mexican American respondents 15 to 44 years of age, in need of family planning services, and not contracepting, was 40; the percentage for Anglos was 35.

290. *Torres A ; Singh S. Hispanic adolescents and contraception. ·Paper presented at the Annual Meeting of the American Public Health Association, Washington, D.C. November 17-21, 1985.

Over the past decade there has been increasing interest in adolescent sexuality, childbearing, pregnancy and contraceptive use. While these issues are well documented for white and black adolescents, there is little data on Hispanic teenagers. This paper analyzes data from the 1982 National Survey of Family Growth to describe the contraceptive experience among this population, and compares it to the experience of white and black non-Hispanics of comparable age. An analysis of age at first intercourse, contraceptive methods used and sources of contraceptive services obtained is also presented. Wherever the sample allows, contraceptive use patterns are analyzed by age (younger and older teens and adult women), marital and poverty status and Hispanic origin.

291. *U.S. Department of Health and Human Services, Centers for Disease Control. Assessment of family planning: United States/ Mexico border. **Morbidity and Mortality Weekly Report.** 1980 Apr; 29(16):181-3.

Data are presented on contraceptive use for Anglos and Hispanics in the four border states of Texas, New Mexico, Arizona and California. Between July and September 1979, the Centers for Disease Control interviewed 2,135 women 15 to 44 years of age from a sample of 5,005 households in 51 border area counties in which 25% or more households had a Hispanic (**Mexican**) head at the time of the 1970 census. Contraceptive use was higher for Anglo respondents than for Hispanics in the three marital status categories: currently, previously and never married. Sterilization and oral contraceptives were the predominant methods among both Anglo and Hispanic respondents. Among currently married Anglo and Hispanic women about equal proportions had been sterilized, but 18% of currently married Anglo men had been sterilized compared to four percent of currently married Hispanic men. Seventy-four percent of never married Anglos and 87% of never married Hispanics were not currently using contraception. Oral contraception was the predominant method for both

Anglo and Hispanic never married women who were using contraception.

292.   *U.S. Department of Health and Human Services,   National
Center for Health Statistics. Contraceptive utilization: United
States, 1976. By: Mosher WP. **Vital and Health Statistics.** 1981
Mar;23(7). 58 p.

This study presents final revised data from Cycle II of the
National Survey of Family Growth, 1976.   Forty-nine percent of
married couples with wives of reproductive age were using non-
surgical contraceptive methods in 1976, and 19% of couples were
using surgical contraceptors.   Of those not using it, 11% were
sterile, 13% pregnant, postpartum or seeking pregnancy, and
eight percent not using it for other reasons.   Distribution of
contraceptive methods changed in important ways over the previous four years.   The number of married women using oral contraceptives dropped from 6.7 to 6.2 million, although it remained
the most popular non-surgical method, accounting for 46% of non-
surgical contraceptors.   Other methods, in descending order of
popularity were condom, IUD, rhythm, foam, diaphragm, and other
methods (such as douche or withdrawal).   Non-surgical methods
were more prevalent where the wife was 15 to 29 years of age;
sterilization more prevalent among those with wives 30 to 44.
Oral contraceptive use was more likely, and use of condom or
diaphragm less likely, among the younger group. Hispanics were
most likely to use the IUD.

293.   *Warren CW ; Smith JC ; Garcia Nunez J ; Rochat RW ;
Martinez-Manautou J. Contraceptive use and family planning ser-
vices along the United States/Mexico border. **International
Family Planning Perspectives.** 1981 Jun;7(2):52-9.

Investigators from the United States Centers for Disease Control
and the Mexican Social Security Institute report on contraceptive use and the unmet need for family planning services along
the border, based on a 1979 survey.   Results show that 75% of
Anglo women (white, non-Hispanic) and 65% of Hispanic women
living on the U.S. side are currently using contraceptives,
while about 50% of the women on the **Mexican** side are current
users.   About 30% of the Mexican women are in need of family
planning services: married, not pregnant, seeking pregnancy, or
sterile, and not using any method of contraception. The comparable level of unmet need among women on the U.S. side is two
percent among Anglos and ten percent among Hispanics.   Mexican
women are somewhat more likely to depend on medical methods
(sterilization, pill, IUD, and injectables) than are Anglo or
other Hispanic women (83%, 76%, and 72%, respectively).   About
one-fifth of the women who use a method opt for sterilization.
Sterilization of the male partner is popular among Anglo couples
(24%), but not among other Hispanics (six percent) or Mexicans
(less than one percent).   Levels of contraceptive use among the
Mexican and other Hispanic women rise with level of education,
but there is little variation among Anglo women on this variable.

294.   *Warren CW ; Smith JC ; Rochat RW. Differentials in the
planning status of most recent live births to Mexican Americans
and Anglos. **Public Health Reports.** 1983 Mar/Apr;98(2):152-60.

Data from personal interviews with 705 **Mexican** American and 363
Anglo women during the 1979 United States/Mexico Border Survey

were analyzed in an effort to answer the following questions:
to what extent was the distribution of most recent live births
that were planned, mistimed, or unwanted different for Mexican
Americans and Anglos; to what extent were differences between
Mexican Americans and Anglos in unwanted births associated with
differences in the distribution of age, parity, education, and
poverty status in these two ethnic groups; and were Mexican
Americans and Anglos whose most recent live birth was unwanted
equally likely to have used contraception before the pregnancy.
Forty-eight percent of the most recent live births to Mexican
Americans were planned; 37% were mistimed, and 15% were unwanted.   Eighteen percent of the most recent births to young
women 15 to 19 years old were planned. As parity increased, the
proportion of most recent live births that were unwanted also
increased.   The use of contraception at the time of conception
was examined for each woman whose most recent live birth was
unwanted. Results showed that 68% of such Anglo women, but only
23% of such Mexican American women, were using contraception at
the time of conception.

3. Sterilization

295. Barron E ; Richardson JA. Counseling women for tubal sterilization. **Health and Social Work.** 1978 Feb;3(1):48-58.

In view of the current concern about sterilization abuse, the federal government has issued guidelines to prevent women from being sterilized without their knowledge or consent. The New York City Health and Hospital Corporation established guidelines that were more stringent still. The revised guidelines demanded that the woman and an auditor/witness of her choice meet with a non-physician counselor and, particularly important in view of the large number of Hispanics interested in the procedure, that all communication be readily understandable and in the patient's primary language. The authors describe a counseling program in a large inner city hospital that followed these specifications. There was a marked ethnic difference among the women who finally decided on the operation; a higher proportion of **Puerto Rican** women accepted the operation than did blacks. In addition, the statistics showed that after the orientation, over one-third of the women changed their minds and decided not to undergo the operation. Not only was the group approach efficient, but a further advantage was that it allowed women to share their concerns among themselves and to learn from one another as well as from professionals.

296. Daily EF ; Nicholas N. Tubal ligations on general service patients seen by peer level family planning counselors in thirty New York City voluntary and municipal hospitals. **American Journal of Obstetrics and Gynecology.** 1975 Nov;123(6):656-9.

From July 1969 to September 1974, 185,927 obstetric/gynecologic and 87,989 abortion patients were seen by peer level counselors selected, trained, and employed full time or part time by the New York City Department of Health's Maternity, Infant Care, Family Planning Projects. The counselors are instructed never to recommend a sterilization procedure unless a patient states she and her husband do not wish more children, at which time the pros and cons of sterilization by vasectomy or tubal ligation are discussed. Obstetric/gynecologic patients having a tubal ligation increased from six percent in 1969 to a high of seven percent in 1972, then declined to five percent during the first nine months of 1974.   Abortion patients requesting tubal ligation remained at two percent during 1970-72, then decreased to one percent during 1974. **Puerto Rican** or Spanish background obstetric patients request almost three times as many ligations as black women and almost six times as many as white women. Similarly, Puerto Rican or other Spanish background abortion patients request and receive tubal ligations at a rate double that of both black and white women.

297. Hunter K ; Linn MW ; Stein SR. Sterilization among American Indian and Chicano mothers. **International Quarterly of Community Health Education.** 1983/84;4(4):343-52.

In a large study of family size and birth control among women from five cultures in the Miami, Florida area, it was noted that 60% of the Miccosukee and Seminole Indians having five or more children were surgically sterile. Whites, however, had a 30% incidence rate and a similar socioeconomic group of Chicanos (**Mexicans**) had a 20% incidence rate. Analyses considered both pre and post-operative differences between the Indians and a comparison group of Chicanos. Though significant cultural differences between the women existed, these had no significant role in predicting sterilization. Factors which may have contributed to the greater incidence of tubal ligation among Indian women are explored. Since low socioeconomic status, poor education or low income may have been influential factors, these variables were controlled by comparison of similar groups. The only factor which might have affected the results so significantly was that on the average, Indian women were four years older than Chicano women. A study of the groups, matched for age, however, indicates an even higher incidence of sterilization for Indian women.

298. Mumford SD. Who elects vasectomy? In: Mumford, SD. **Vasectomy counseling.** San Francisco, California, San Francisco Press. 1977. p. 6-15.

People of all socioeconomic groups elect vasectomy if there are no barriers, particularly economic and eligibility. The economic barrier faced by hundreds of thousands of men in the United States who desire vasectomy determines to some extent who elects vasectomy. At the Houston Clinic there is no such barrier, for the vasectomy is free of charge for those who cannot pay the $75 fee. In sum, the best answer to the question who elects vasectomy? is people who desire no more children, representing all socioeconomic subgroups in numbers that would be expected if vasectomy were a random event, with one exception. This exception is that the numbers of **Mexican** Americans and of blacks are disproportionately small compared with whites. Formal education, income, occupation, marital status, years married, employment status, religious preference, and number of children have little influence on men (as a group) with respect to electing vasectomy. A majority of the men who choose vasectomy are not in desperate circumstances. They are instead faced with circumstances that make the vasectomy strictly elective. Men who choose vasectomy almost always have discussed vasectomy with a trusted vasectomized man.

299. Petchesky RP. Reproductive choice in the contemporary United States: a social analysis of female sterilization. In:

Michaelson KL, ed. **And the poor get children: radical perspectives on population dynamics.** New York City, Monthly Review
Press. 1981. p. 50-88.

Sterilization patterns vary among different groups of women,
illustrating   that broad social conditions and   structured   inequalities,   rather than individual preferences or technology determine women's birth control experience.   According to one
study, based on data from the National Survey of Family Growth,
sterilization in the United States is currently the most popular
contraceptive method for all married couples.   Rates are significantly higher   among low income women and women of little
education   than among middle income and college educated women.
There are differences in sex and ethnic patterns of   sterilization.   Among   most minority groups, women rather than men are
sterilized.   Among white and middle class married couples there
is a high proportion of vasectomies.   Black, Hispanic, and
Native American women are more likely than white women to be the
victims of involuntary sterilization or hysterectomy for contraceptive purposes.   The increases in sterilizations represents
very different realities for different groups, reflecting the
major divisions of class, race, and sex.   Like birth rates,
rates of sterilization among different social groups cannot be
compared apart from their social context.

300.   Schensul   SL ; Borrero M ; Barrera V ; Backstrand J ;
Guarnaccia P.   A model of fertility control in a Puerto Rican
community. **Urban Anthropology.** 1982 Spring;11(1):81-99.

This   article examines the fertility control decision-making of
Puerto Rican women in Hartford, Connecticut, a city that has a
high sterilization rate among Puerto Rican heads or co-heads of
households.   A survey of 153 female household heads in Hartford,
conducted in 1978-79 by the Hispanic Health Council, found that
79 (52%) had been sterilized.   The results indicate that Puerto
Rican women begin their sexual activity with limited use of
birth control, accept reversible methods primarily after the
second and third births, become sterilized in significant numbers after their third child, and have generally attained sterilization after five births.   Sterilization is the fertility
control method most frequently selected at the point where women
feel they have reached their desired family size. Since optimal
family size is achieved quickly, many Puerto Rican women seek
sterilization in their 20s. This widespread acceptance of sterilization in part reflects the effects of recent sterilization
campaigns in Puerto Rico.   It further reflects health care
providers' expectation that Puerto Rican women will not be
successful in their use of reversible methods.

301. Scrimshaw SC ; Pasquariella B. An exploratory study of
variables associated with the acceptance of female sterilization
in Spanish Harlem. Paper presented at the American Association
of Planned Parenthood Physicians Eighth Annual Meeting, Boston,
Massachusetts. April, 1970. 22 p.

A group of sterilized women and a group of non-sterilized women
were interviewed in Spanish Harlem in the summer of 1969.   The
sterilized group consists of women who considered sterilization
a convenient and secure way to avoid pregnancy.   Most used it
to limit their family size before it became excessively large.
Nearly two-thirds of the non-sterilized women said they would
accept sterilization in the future, despite the difficulty in

obtaining the operation, the opposition of the Catholic church, and the availability of other contraceptive methods. There is a demand for sterilization, particularly among **Puerto Ricans**, which is poorly met at present due primarily to restrictive hospital policies and ambivalence on the part of physicians. It is clear that the role of female sterilization in family planning has potential significance, and must be considered more fully than it has been in the past.

302. *Scrimshaw SC ; Pasquariella B. Variables associated with the demand for female sterilization in Spanish Harlem. New York International Institute for the Study of Human Reproduction, Division for Program Development and Evaluation. January, 1970. 73 p.

In this study interviews were obtained from 40 sterilized and 51 non-sterilized women from Spanish Harlem in New York City. The actual mean family size was 4.7, ideal mean family size 3.1 for sterilized women, and 2.4 and 2.6 respectively for non-sterilized women. Ninety-five percent of the sterilized women, and 71% of the others were **Puerto Rican**; five percent and 28% were blacks. Blacks prefer to rely on the pill or IUD and express fears of sterilization, while Puerto Ricans tend to distrust the pill and IUD and prefer sterilization. It appears that some Puerto Ricans are going directly to sterilization rather than trying contraceptives first. Twenty-three percent of the sterilized women had been sterilized while living in Puerto Rico, 18% had gone to Puerto Rico from New York to be sterilized and 60% had been operated on in New York. Sixty-five percent of the operations had been done postpartum. Convenience was given by 75% of the women as their reason for choosing sterilization. Sixty-seven percent cited concern over family size and 50% cited medical reasons.

303. *Vaughan D ; Sparer G. Ethnic group and welfare status of women ·sterilized in federally funded family planning programs: 1972. **Family Planning Perspectives.** 1974 Fall;6(4):224-9.

This study uses data from the National Reporting System for Family Planning Services (NRSFPS), to address the following question: other things being equal, were women from minority groups and women receiving public assistance more likely to be sterilized than other women in federally assisted family planning projects covered by NRSFPS? It examines the data from projects which reported at least 20 sterilization patients of either sex during the year 1972 (a total of 101 family planning projects covering approximately 550,000 women). The data are sufficient to demonstrate that, within the study projects, women of Latin American descent and black women are not disproportionately represented among those electing contraceptive sterilization when age and parity are controlled. Among whites, the same can be said, generally, with regard to welfare recipients as compared to non-recipients; there is insufficient data to indicate whether the same is true for women of Latin American descent. Among non-whites, the data suggest that welfare recipients have about one-third more sterilizations than non-recipients even when age and parity are controlled.

304. Warren CW ; Smith JC ; Rochat RW ; Holck SE. Contraceptive sterilization: a comparison between Mexican Americans and Anglos living in United States counties bordering Mexico. **Social Biology.** 1981 Fall/Winter;28(3/4):265-80.

Prior   to the United States/Mexico Border Survey of Maternal and
Child Health and Family Planning conducted by the Centers for
Disease Control in 1979, little information was available concerning the extent to which **Mexican** Americans in the U.S.,
relative to Anglos, were using male and female sterilization for
contraceptive reasons.   This paper focuses on the comparison of
the two groups in terms of: 1) the prevalence of contraceptive
sterilization; 2) the social and demographic characteristics of
users of contraceptive sterilization; and 3) the timing during
tne reproductive life cycle when contraceptive sterilization
occurs.   For both Mexican Americans and Anglos, contraceptive
sterilization (male and female) was the second most prevalent
method used.   Anglos were more likely to use male than female
sterilization (22% versus 20%), while Mexican Americans were
much more likely to use female than male sterilization (23%
versus six percent).   Having an unwanted last live birth and/or
high parity were important factors related to use of female
sterilization for both Mexican Americans and Anglos.

PART FOUR
CONSEQUENCES OF CHILDBEARING

1. Programs and Consequences for Adolescent Parents

Most of the data on the consequences of early childbearing for Hispanic adolescents come from small studies or evaluations of programs for teen parents. The consequences examined include such things as **educational attainment, labor force participation, self-esteem, readiness for parenthood, child development, attachment to and interaction with children, utilization of health services, receipt of family support, life stress and attitudes toward childrearing.** School return and graduation have received particular attention since Hispanics have substantially higher dropout rates than other United States adolescents even before considering the additional risks due to early parenthood.

Studies which shed light on the general consequences of fertility for Hispanic adults have measured such variables as the **incidence of low birth weight infants,** other measures of child health status, **childrearing attitudes, labor force participation, postpartum depression, family support and attitudes toward newborn infants.**

305. *Berkman-Sherry L. Health care patterns of teenage mothers and their young children. Doctoral Dissertation, Los Angeles, California, University of California. 1980. 280 p. DAI;41(4-A): 1773.

The influence of age on the use of health care services was examined with data on attitudes towards health care and care professionals, knowledge of medical concepts, and use of health services gathered from teenage and non-teenage mothers. The responses of white, black, and **Mexican** American mothers were examined. The mother's age was found to be directly related to years of schooling and presence of older children in the home, and inversely related to household income, work experience, and the presence of adult relatives in the home. Ethnicity provided an influence on attitudes, knowledge and utilization of health services. Age was found to be relevant only in terms of lay care use and preferred informational resources. Teenage mothers

were less likely to use home remedies and over the counter
medications than non-teenage mothers, and were more likely to
rely upon relatives for health care information.   Results indicate no age related differences in the use of health services or
in orientations toward use of medical professionals.

306.   *Brown SV.   Early childbearing and poverty: implications
for social services. **Adolescence.** 1982 Summer;17(66):397-408.

Economic problems are among the most adverse consequences associated with early childbearing.   This paper looks at various
social services to determine whether current services are assisting teenage mothers who live at or below the poverty line to
move toward greater productivity and self-sufficiency in adult-
hood.   The results of a national survey of public social services to teenage mothers show that not only are current services
inadequate, but are lacking in areas which are directly related
to the future economic well being of early childbearing females.
Public social services appear to be ineffectual in alleviating
the conditions that lead to poverty, namely deficits connected
with education, employment, home management and family planning.
Black and Hispanic teenage mothers were found to be at highest
risk of poverty conditions due to their greater dependence on
public agencies.   The implications of these service deficiencies
are discussed in relation to the future economic welfare of
these teenage mothers and the need for a restructuring of social
services in the traditional child welfare sector.

307.   *Cannon-Bonventre K ; Kahn J.   Interviews with adolescent
parents. **Children Today.** 1979 Sep/Oct;8(5):17-9.

Over 100 black, white and Hispanic parents aged 16 to 19 at
delivery were interviewed in the Boston area about their problems and experiences as parents.   The majority were low income;
three-quarters of the mothers reported an annual income of less
than $4,000.   Over one-third of the fathers received public
assistance.   Help from family was also important, and one-third
of the mothers had paid employment.   About three-quarters of the
mothers were married, and 68% had only one child. Although 60%
of the mothers reported having felt very ready for parenthood at
the time of their pregnancy, only 42% felt they actually were
"very ready."   About half reported having less freedom and more
responsibility since becoming parents.   The problems of young
parents are similar to those encountered by people who delay
childbearing, but appear to be exacerbated by youth and lack of
experience.   Shortage of financial resources was the most frequently reported problem, followed by isolation and loneliness.
Location of dependable and acceptable child care and completion
of schooling were other frequently experienced problems.   The
study disclosed a number of areas in which the perspectives of
young parents and service providers were at odds, and made
several recommendations for improved services for young parents.

308.   *Chung HC ; Sibirsky S.   Needs, goals, and programs for
adolescent Hispanic parents in Connecticut. Prepared for Hispanic Policy Development, Washington, D.C., University of Bridgeport, The Urban Management Institute. 1984. 34 p.

In 1982-83, the Urban Management Institute of the University of
Bridgeport surveyed 500 Hispanic households with 1,876 members
residing in Connecticut.   It was the first survey of its kind to
generate detailed socioeconomic and demographic characteristics

of the rapidly growing Hispanic population in Connecticut.   As
of 1983, of 136,000 Hispanic people in Connecticut, (more than
70% of whom were **Puerto Ricans**), 18,000 (13%) were between the
ages of 16 and 21.   Of these, roughly 3,500, or one out of five
youths, were adolescent parents.   The majority of these 3,500
were young mothers who had to raise their children without their
spouses present.   This may mean as high as two out of five
female Hispanic youths had their own children.   It was also
estimated that over 60% of Hispanic parents between ages 16 and
19 had out-of-wedlock children.   The percentage was approximately 50% for the 16 to 21 age group.   Teenage birth and non-
teenage birth mothers and their husbands are compared in terms
of number of children, school dropout and grades completed,
place of birth, English proficiency and labor force participation.   Teenage birth parents were at a relative disadvantage on
all measures.

309. *Garcia Coll CT. The consequences of teenage childbearing
in traditional Puerto Rican culture. To appear in: Nugent L,
Lester BM, and Brazelton TB, eds. **Cultural context of infancy.**
New Jersey, Ablex. 1985. 35 p.

The high risk factors associated with teenage childbearing are
reviewed in this paper.   A cross-cultural study was done using
30 primiparous women in Puerto Rico, and 30 primiparous women in
Providence, Rhode Island.   All the American women were Caucasian.   Data were collected on social support, life stress, and
maternal attitudes toward rearing a child.   Adolescent mothers
from Puerto Rico expected more frequent help from their support
network than any other group.   They report relying more on peers
than on adults for child care support, especially the child's
father.   Adolescent mothers from Providence reported having more
life events within the last year, supporting the conceptualiza-
tion of pregnancy during adolescence as a more stressful event
within this culture than in **Puerto Rican** culture. No major
differences in maternal attitudes between adolescent and older
mothers were found.   However, Puerto Rican mothers reported
lower maternal satisfaction, maternal moderation of the child's
aggressive challenge, maternal flexibility, and encouragement of
positive interaction with the child.   Whether these differences
are determined by culture or by socioeconomic status is not
known.   Puerto Rican mothers reported more positive beliefs
around teenage childbearing than mothers in Providence.   Findings support the notion that the cultural context of adolescent
childbearing within a low socioeconomic status, urban Puerto
Rican population is, in comparison, supportive and positive.
This is not to imply that early childbearing is the best option
for these women.

310. *Haggstrom GW ; Blaschke TJ ; Kanouse DE ; Lisowski W ;
Morrison PA. Teenage parents: their ambitions and attainments.
Prepared for the National Institute of Child Health and Human
Development, National Institute of Health, Santa Monica, Cali-
fornia, Rand Corporation. 1981. 239 p.

The research is based on the National Longitudinal Study of the
High School Class of 1973 (NLS), the more than 22,000 participants of which were the subjects of follow-up surveys in 1973,
1974, and 1976.   Tables include data on race, ethnicity, region,
socioeconomic status, and family background.   Measurements of
academic aptitude and scholastic performance, taken before the
participants had graduated, reveal that those who soon became

parents ranked lower in these areas and in socioeconomic status than did their classmates.   Thus, preexisting differences would have led to different outcomes even in the absence of parent- hood.   Analysis also reveals that many of the adverse conse- quences attributed to early parenthood also showed up among those who married early but remained childless.   Married women who became mothers early displayed a shift in career and educa- tional goals and achievements, and those who entered the labor market received considerably lower wages than non-mothers. Single mothers rely heavily on families and society for finan- cial support.   The NLS excludes those who became parents during early adolescence and those who dropped out of school before graduation.

311. *Haggstrom GW ; Morrison PA. Investigating adolescent parenthood with the National Longitudinal Study of High School Seniors. Rand Paper Series, Rand Corporation. February, 1979.

This paper is an interim report on a study of adolescent parent- hood.   The research is based on a large panel study known as the National Longitudinal Study of the High School Class of 1972 (NLS), which has traced over 22,000 adolescents who are now in their early 20s and have experienced many of the near term consequences of early parenthood.   Three areas of endeavor are treated.   First described are procedures for creating variables that mark entry into marriage and commencement of parenthood for the NLS respondents, thereby rectifying serious deficiencies in the NLS data base.   The technical discussion of these proce- dures is intended primarily for other researchers who may want to adopt the procedures in working with the same data set. Second, the authors provide a descriptive profile of four cate- gories of respondents: late adolescent parents, early adult parents, adult parents, and non-parents. This profile affords interesting descriptive comparisons among parents and non- parents, as well as certain benchmark comparisons for validation purposes.   Third, a statistical model is developed for gauging the consequences of early parenthood. This model addresses cer- tain methodological issues in assessing consequences from data sets that contain data for both parents and non-parents.

312. *Held L. Self-esteem and social network of the young pregnant teenager. **Adolescence**. 1981 Winter;16(64):905-12.

Annually, 250,000 women 17 years of age and younger, become pregnant.   Nevertheless, psychosocial factors involved in teen- age pregnancies are not well documented.   The self-esteem and social networks of 62 black, white, and **Mexican** American women, 17 years of age and under, were examined in this study.   The Coopersmith Self-Esteem Inventory was used to determine per- ceived levels of self-esteem.   Social networks were explored by asking the subjects to rate their perceptions of reactions to their pregnancy by significant others.   The subjects were then asked to rank these significant others in order of their impor- tance. Future plans were also surveyed.   Of the significant others, mothers of the subjects were most disapproving of the pregnancy, whereas the father of the baby was perceived as being most approving.   Mothers of the subjects were more often ranked as being most important to the subjects than other significant others.   Pregnant black women were more likely to be in school or planning to return to school than white or Mexican Americans.

313. *Levy SB ; Grinker WJ. Choices and life circumstances: an

ethnographic study of Project Redirection teens. Manpower Demonstration Research Corporation. June, 1983.

This paper presents the results of an ethnographic study of a sample of participants of Project Redirection, a program for teenage mothers with sites in Phoenix, Arizona; Riverside, Massachusetts; and Harlem in New York. Ethnic differences in sexual activity, education, employment and career aspirations, marriage, and family networks of the participants are examined. There appeared to be little cultural difference among the blacks, whites and Chicanos (**Mexicans**) in attitudes toward premarital sex. Overall Chicano teens were not as inclined to complete school as were the black and white participants, and were more likely to look to marriage and not a career as a means of future support. Many mothers of black teens were themselves single parents who were employed full time and thus had difficulty assisting their daughters with child care. The typical Chicana mother was at home where child care assistance could more easily be provided. Yet it was more frequently the black parent who strongly encouraged her daughter's return to school. The implications of the findings for planning teen pregnancy programs are discussed.

314. *Martinez AL. The impact of adolescent pregnancy on Hispanic adolescents and their families. In: Ooms T, ed. **Teenage pregnancy in a family context: implications for policy.** Philadelphia, Pennsylvania, Temple University Press. 1981. p. 326-44.

Although Hispanics in the United States are not a homogeneous population, many cultural, linguistic, and traditional values are held in common. The slow but generally continuous contact that occurs between Hispanics in the U.S. and relatives from Latin America acts as a protector and promoter of values, among them sexual values, that differ from the current values in the U.S. Studies must be performed which address the following questions: 1) what are the causes of adolescent sexual behavior among Hispanic young people within their cultural context? 2) what are the consequences of this behavior in terms of education, health, economic, and social status? 3) how do the differing cultural attitudes regarding sexual behavior and expectations affect Hispanic young people? 4) what are the relationships between Hispanic unemployment, school dropout, drug or alcohol use, and adolescent sexual behavior? 5) what are the prevailing attitudes toward abortion among Hispanic young people, compared to practice? 6) what are the immediate and long term effects of early parenting and/or marriage on these young people? 7) what percentage of women of Hispanic origin have children; what is their age breakdown; what are their national origins? 8) to what extent are Hispanic families changing or moving away from extended families?

315. *Mosena PW. Adolescent parent outreach follow-up study. University of Chicago, Children's Policy Research Project. 1985.

A great deal is known about the demographics, determinants and consequences of adolescent childbearing in the United States. In contrast, very little is known about the dynamics of adolescent parenthood, how do the needs and desires of teenage mothers change over time and under specific conditions as their children move from infancy into childhood. This gap is particularly true for the most dependent portion of the teenage parent population, those on Aid to Families with Dependent Children

(AFDC).   This report presents findings from the Adolescent Parent Outreach Survey, a longitudinal study of young mothers on
AFDC in Cook County, Illinois.   Eight hundred and ninety nine
white, black and Hispanic welfare mothers under age 18, with one
or more children, or pregnant with their first child, were
surveyed.   The purpose was to obtain information about the life
circumstances of these young mothers and their children once
they go on welfare.   Personal and family background characteristics associated with completing high school, and having a second
birth are identified.   Sources of social support are also examined.   Characteristics and social support for the three racial/
ethnic groups are compared.

316.   *Mott FL.   The pace of repeated childbearing among young
American mothers.   **Family Planning Perspectives.** 1986 Jan/Feb;18
(1):5-12.

This study analyzes the pace and determinants of repeat childbearing among a sample of white, black and Hispanic women first
interviewed as part of the National Longitudinal Survey (NLS) in
1979 and reinterviewed in 1983.   The analysis focuses on 1,448
women who had a child at least 24 months prior to the 1983
survey.   Among all women aged 24 and 25 in the NLS, 12% of the
whites had had a birth by age 19, as compared to 35% of the
blacks, and 24% of the Hispanics.   Among the sample of mothers,
the Hispanic women were generally more likely than either the
blacks or the whites to have a second birth soon after the first
(within 24 or 36 months) at nearly every age at first birth.
However, although Hispanic women generally are more likely than
either white or black women to quickly follow-up an early first
birth, the youngest mothers are not significantly more likely
than the oldest mothers to have a second child quickly.   The
findings for Hispanic mothers, who report generally higher fertility expectations and lower educational expectations than do
other mothers, suggest that these women represent a relatively
unacculturated subgroup, with more traditional attitudes toward
motherhood and higher education for women.

317.   *Mott FL ; Marsiglio W. Early childbearing and completion
of high school.   **Family Planning Perspectives.** 1985 Sep/Oct;17
(5):234-7.

This study used data from the National Longitudinal Survey of
Work Experience of Youth to look at the consequences of adolescent parenthood for 4,696 women who were aged 20 to 26 in 1983.
Black women in each childbearing category were about as likely
as white women to have completed high school, but Hispanic women
were less likely to have done so.   Indeed, while completion
rates are only slightly lower for childless Hispanic women (87%)
than for corresponding whites and blacks (95% and 93%), they are
markedly lower for Hispanic women who have become mothers.
Thus, among Hispanic mothers who gave birth shortly after leaving school, the proportion completing their secondary education
is 20 points lower than it is among whites or blacks (33% versus
55%); and among Hispanic mothers who became pregnant after
leaving school, the proportion is nearly 30 points lower (55%
versus 81-85%).   These findings are consistent with the view,
advanced in previous research, that Hispanic women may be influenced by stronger cultural norms regarding separation of the
parent and student roles than are other groups.

318.   *Ortiz V ; Cooney RS. The effect of early marital and

fertility events on the educational attainment of young Hispanic females and non-Hispanic white females. Paper presented at the Population Association of America Annual Meeting, San Diego, California. (Unpublished) April 30, 1982. 33 p.

In comparison to the majority of white youths, Hispanic females have a lower educational attainment, higher fertility rate at younger ages, and come from more disadvantaged socioeconomic backgrounds. The role of socioeconomic characteristics in the lower educational status of Hispanic females is examined. Analysis is based on the Youth Cohort of the Longitudinal Survey of the Labor Market Experience, specifically the first year interviews conducted in 1979, of the five year survey. The cohort of approximately 12,700 youths was sampled to be nationally representative of youths between the ages of 14 and 21. The analysis in this paper is restricted to respondents who are 16 years of age or older. Young women who became pregnant, regardless of whether they had also married or not, completed fewer years of schooling. Those who became pregnant, but did not marry were considerably more likely to drop out of school. Young Hispanic women were just as affected by marrying or having a child at an early age as were women in general. The findings of the study provide strong support for the negative consequences of early marital and fertility events, especially a pregnancy, on educational attainment.

319. *Ortiz V ; Gurak DT. School to work transition: a comparative analysis of Hispanic and white youth. Bronx, New York, Fordham University, Hispanic Research Center. May, 1982.

This research examines the school to work transition of Hispanic youth as compared with non-Hispanic white youth. In addition to comparing Hispanics and whites, further distinctions were made among Hispanics based on ethnicity and generational status. Several studies have demonstrated that marital status and the presence of children are related to participation in the labor force of women in general (Hofferth and Moore, 1979; Mott and Shaw, 1978), and of Hispanic females. Thus, for example, when the focus is on dropping out of high school whether or not a young woman is married and/or pregnant at that time, which can be determined from the detailed history available in the National Longitudinal Survey, will be used as the independent variable. The independent variables also included sex and age. The four major sets of variables were analyzed to explain differences between Hispanics and non-Hispanic whites at critical points in the educational process: dropping out of high school, graduating from high school, but not continuing on to college, and dropping out of college. When focusing on labor force experiences, only respondents who had completed their education were included in the analysis, and educational attainment was included as an independent variable.

320. *Philliber SG ; Darabi KF ; Graham E. Adolescent parenthood. In: Ahmed P, ed. **Pregnancy, childbirth, and parenthood.** New York, Elsevier. 1981. p. 201-9. (Coping with Medical Issues).

This paper describes the perspectives of adolescent mothers on their own experiences with early childbearing. Ninety-three black and Hispanic women who delivered their first children in New York City hospital wards as teenagers in 1975 were interviewed in their homes with their children, who ranged in age

from two and a half to four years old.   The most common change
in their lives mentioned by the young women was a reduction in
the amount of time available to go out or pursue old interests.
Fifteen percent mentioned more specific limitations in relation
to marriage, school, or work.   Some of the women were able to
overcome the restrictions with parental help.   Fourteen percent
mentioned positive changes since the birth of the first child,
most frequently personal growth or maturity.   Other positive
changes mentioned included the love or happiness brought by the
presence of a child.   A slight majority, of both black and
Hispanic teenagers said that their lives had been better since
they became mothers.   Nevertheless, most also stated they
wished their first births had occurred later.   Taken together,
the data appear to cast doubt on the assumption that teenage
parenthood is always a negative experience.

321.   *Philliber SG ; Graham EH. The impact of age of mother on
mother/child interaction patterns. **Journal of Marriage and the
Family**. 1981 Feb;43:109-15.

An investigation of the impact of maternal age on mother and
child interaction patterns was undertaken among 282 urban black
and Hispanic ward patients who gave birth to their first child
in 1975 at a hospital in New York City.   Regression analysis
demonstrating maternal age did not significantly influence
mother and child interaction patterns when other relevant variables were controlled.   These findings did not support the
widely held view that young mothers tend to make poor parents.
Data on 11 independent variables and on six dependent measures
of parent and child interaction were obtained by interviewing
and observing the mothers in their own homes when the children
were two to four years of age.   The children of black women
apparently received more opportunities for daily stimulation
than did the children of Latin women.   Since this scale included
items on presence of relatives and reading to the child, perhaps
the Latin mothers were at a disadvantage because of the absence
of relatives in the area or because of the lesser availability
of books in Spanish.   Factors such as parity, age of the child,
ethnic affiliation, and socioeconomic status were controlled for
by choosing a homogeneous study population.   Twenty-six percent
of the mothers were less than 20 years of age.   Mother's age did
not have an effect on the dependent variables when the other
independent variables were controlled for.

322.   *Polit DF ; Kahn JR.   Early subsequent pregnancy among
economically disadvantaged teenage mothers. **American Journal of
Public Health**. 1986 Feb;78(2):167-71.

This study investigated the antecedents and short term consequences of an early subsequent pregnancy in a sample of economically disadvantaged teenage mothers.   Data were gathered over a
two year period from a sample of 675 young mothers (46% black,
24% Mexican American, 18% Puerto Rican, and nine percent white)
living in eight United States cities.   Within two years of the
initial interview, when half the sample was still pregnant with
the index pregnancy, nearly half of the sample experienced a
second or higher order pregnancy.   Characteristics of the young
women at entry into the study were relatively poor predictors of
which teenagers would conceive again by final interview.   An
early repeat pregnancy was associated with a number of negative
short term consequences in the areas of education, employment,
and welfare dependency, even after background characteristics

were statistically controlled.

323. *Polit DF ; Tannen MB ; Kahn JR. School, work and family
planning: interim impacts in Project Redirection. New York City,
Manpower Demonstration Research Corporation. June, 1983. No.
xxxi, 197 p.

Project Redirection was created in 1980 out of concern for an
issue that has assumed increasing importance on the nation's
agenda: the high rate of teenage pregnancy, particularly among
the disadvantaged.   The programs in Boston, Arizona and California enroll pregnant teenagers and teen mothers under 18 years
of age, without high school diplomas, and for the most part,
living in families receiving welfare. Project Redirection
serves a large Hispanic clientele. Ninety-two percent of the
enrollees in Boston are **Puerto Rican,** 53% and 29% respectively
of those in Phoenix and Riverside are Chicanos (**Mexicans**). This
report discusses evaluation impact findings 12 months after the
teens were enrolled in Project Redirection. Project Redirection participants experienced a significantly lower rate of post
baseline pregnancies (17%) than the comparison group teens
(22%). Hispanic teens in the program were less likely than
blacks or whites to be in school at follow-up, but more likely
to have worked. They also had the lowest educational aspirations at the 12 month interview. However, Hispanics were not
significantly more likely to have had a repeat pregnancy and no
ethnic differences were found in birth control knowledge scores
at follow-up.

324. *Rogeness GA ; Ritchey S ; Alex PL ; Zuelzer M ; Morris R.
Family- patterns and parenting attitudes in teenage parents.
Journal of Community Psychology. 1981;9(3):239-45.

A group of 55 primarily **Mexican** American teenage mothers were
interviewed and compared with 45 never pregnant teenagers attending a local high school and 20 never pregnant teenagers
attending a mental health clinic. A Support System Questionnaire was developed to obtain information on whom the teenager
saw as helpful in her environment and to gain information on
some of her attitudes and future goals. The Michigan Screening
Profile of Parenting was developed to help identify parents and
potential parents who are at risk, especially for child abuse.
The teen parents grew up and were currently living in significantly more single parent families than the high school group.
The teen parent and clinic groups were similar in the percent
who grew up in single parent families, the percent currently
living with the biological father in the home, and their desired
family size, even though the two groups were markedly different
in economic and ethnic background. The teen parent and clinic
groups both had a significantly higher likelihood of a problem
in the relationship with their parents than did the high school
group. The teen parent group was different from the other two
groups in that more members were isolated, less interested in
obtaining new information, and less oriented toward work and
school.

325. Rothenberg PB ; Varga PE. The relationship between age of
mother and child health and development. **American Journal of
Public Health.** 1981 Aug;71(8):810-7.

This study investigates the relationship between age of mother
and children's health and development at birth and at approxi-

mately three years of age.   The sample is composed of black and
Hispanic women and their first born children who were delivered
on the wards of a large New York City hospital in 1975.   There
were   no differences between children of teenage and older
mothers in terms of prematurity or birth weight, but the children of younger mothers had higher Apgar scores than those of
older mothers.   Age of mother was not significantly related to
hospitalizations, the need to see a physician regularly,   or
abnormal weight.   Although the number of injurious conditions
and the incidence of burns were higher among the children of
adolescent mothers, the effect of age of mother was not independent of other factors.   The children of teenage mothers scored
better than those of older mothers on the total Denver Developmental Screening Test, as well as on the Fine Motor   sector.
These findings thus suggest that when relevant background characteristics are controlled, children of teenage mothers are as
healthy and develop as well as children of older mothers.

326. *Takai RT ; Owings JA. In and out of school consequences
of adolescent parenthood: evidence from High School and Beyond.
Paper presented at the American Educational Research Association
Annual Meeting, Montreal, Canada. 1983.

The purpose of this paper is to examine the consequences of
adolescent parenthood at two critical points, sophomore   and
senior years of high school.   The analysis uses data from the
first two waves of an NCES study, High School and Beyond,   a
nationally representative sample of 1,980 high school sophomores
and seniors in the United States.   Analyzing longitudinal data
has shown that the effects of early entry into parenthood on
several outcome measures differs for males and females.   Having
a child is positively related to dropping out of school   and
negatively related to educational expectations for females, but
not for males.   Black and Hispanic sophomores are more likely
than white students to have higher 1982 occupational plans and
expectations.   However, in a multivariate model Hispanic sophomore females were not significantly more likely than whites to
leave high school before graduation.

327. *Teberg AJ ; Howell VV ; Wingert WA. Attachment interaction behavior between young teenage mothers and their infants.
Journal of Adolescent Health Care. 1983;4(1):61-6.

Behavioral interaction between teenage mothers and their infants
is explored in this paper. Twenty-six low income level Hispanic
teenage mothers (mean age 15 years) and their infants (mean age
13.5 months) were compared with an older control group of 30
mothers (mean age 26 years) and their infants (mean age 14
months).   Infant attachment, exploration, and stress adaptation
behaviors and maternal ability to contact, encourage, and com-
fort the infant are evaluated.   Twenty-six percent of the control infants show limited ability to cope with stress compared
to 47% of infants of teenage mothers.   Control mothers differ
significantly from teenage mothers in effective eye, verbal,
physical contact, and smiling behaviors.   These findings suggest that limited teenage maternal behaviors may potentially
have a negative psychological effect for both infants and their
young mothers.

328. *Testa M. The social support of adolescent parents: a
survey of young mothers on Aid to Families with Dependent Children in Illinois. Chicago, Illinois, University of Chicago,

NORC, Children's Policy Research Project. (Unpublished) 1985.

This report is an analysis of a social survey of mothers under 18 years of age who are recipients of the government's Aid to Families with Dependent Children (AFDC) in the State of Illinois. The statewide sample of 1,909 young mothers included 627 whites, 1,032 blacks, and 250 Hispanics. The study aimed to present the consequences of adolescent parenthood for AFDC recipients and the findings are organized by the topical areas of family support, school, work, health, contraception, and second pregnancies. Significant differences in the experiences, goals and needs across the various subgroups are presented according to race, ethnicity, family background, and geography. Included is a comprehensive examination of adolescent parenthood among Hispanics.

329. *Welti VS. Adolescent pregnancy and motherhood: a case study investigation. Doctoral Dissertation, Berkeley, California, California School of Professional Psychology. 1975. 251 p. DAI;36(8-B):4186.

Three adolescents who became pregnant out-of-wedlock and kept and raised their children were studied to determine their mothering capabilities. Subjects were white, black and Mexican American girls from the upper/lower class. A case study approach was utilized to investigate the personal, social, and environmental variables within the lives of the three subjects which affected their abilities to mother their children. Effective mothering was conceptualized in terms of a mother's acceptance of her child. Mothering adequacy was determined by observing and examining each adolescent's interaction with her child within the parameters of acceptance or non-acceptance behavior. The study determined that in the case of adolescent pregnancy, it is possible to predict outcomes for the mother and her child based on an examination of an adolescent's personality dynamics, the psychological meaning of the pregnancy for her, and her personal, social, and environmental support system. Implications of the study are discussed, and suggestions are made for comprehensive programs to deal with the present and future problems that adolescent pregnancy and motherhood present.

330. *Young WR III. New Mexico dropout study: 1979-1980. Santa Fe, New Mexico, State Department of Education, Evaluation, Assessment and Testing Unit. 1981.

The study for 1979-80 identified 8,414 or nine percent of the statewide enrollment of 91,438 for grades nine through 12, as school dropouts, using surveys tallying all dropouts and enrollment by grade, sex, ethnicity, school, district, and possible reasons for leaving school, from 144 schools in 86 districts. The lowest rate was for grade nine, the highest for grade 11, typical of the previous three years. Also consistent with past results was a higher dropout rate for males (ten percent) than females (nine percent), although the differential was less. Major causes for dropping out for both males and females were motivational and interest related (41% and 32% respectively), and home or related (16% and 27% respectively). Further analysis attributed the 27% rate for females to pregnancy or marriage. Anglos, Hispanics and blacks had similar ranges (eight percent, nine percent, nine percent), with an increase for Native Americans (14%). Anglos and Hispanics dropped out most

in grade 11, Native Americans in grade ten, and blacks in grade
12, with the major causes for all groups reported as motivational or interest related.   Five schools and three districts
had no dropouts.   Included in the report are the survey, data
tabulation, and a map showing dropout rates by school district.

2. Fertility Consequences for Adults

331. Bean FD ; Swicegood CG ; King AG. Fertility and labor supply among Hispanic American women. Austin, Texas, University of Texas, Texas Population Research Center. 1982. 34 p. (Texas Population Research Center Paper No. 3.017).

Focus in this paper is on the fertility labor supply relation-ship among groups of **Mexican** American, **Cuban** American, and **Puerto Rican** women. The analyses are based on data from the 1976 Survey of Income and Education. The nature of the labor markets to which these women might have access was indexed by their English proficiency, generational status, education and husband's income levels. The role incompatibility hypothesis directs attention to the interaction of these variables with the various measures of fertility. Also considered were the effects of household composition variables which record the presence of older children and non-parental adults in the household as a factor which lessens the constraint of fertility on female labor supply. The results indicate that these variables were signifi-cant in their interactions with fertility, particularly among Mexican Americans, but the signs of the effects were not always in the expected direction among Cuban Americans. Cuban Ameri-cans seemed to be less deterred by the presence of children, the higher the socioeconomic status, and the greater the English proficiency, but the anomalous results for the Cuban American women were based on such a small number of cases that not too much significance should be given to them.

332. Boulette TR. Parenting: special needs of low income Spanish surnamed families. **Pediatric Annals.** 1977 Sep;6(9):613-9.

Intervention strategies with the low income Spanish speaking or Spanish surnamed population must be based on the reality that we currently know very little about their core culture, family, and childrearing values and practices. The intervening influences of prejudice, social class, nativity, biculturation, family differences, and presence of physical and mental pathology must also be considered. Inappropriate generalizations derived from poorly designed studies, anecdotal reports of isolated enclaves, authors' romantic or deprecatory prejudices, and reports of the victim's acceptance of stereotypes are the essence of our current knowledge. The pediatrician or family counselor must avoid cultural generalizations if he hopes to work effectively with these families. Instead, the practitioner must consider individual cultural values and practices and the poverty specific concomitants that can influence child care.

333. *Engle PL ; Scrimshaw SC ; Smidt R. Sex differences in attitudes towards newborn infants among women of Mexican origin. **Medical Anthropology.** 1984 Spring;8(2):133-44.

This paper analyzes a data set on women of **Mexican** origin delivering in Los Angeles hospitals in order to examine whether Mexican women's attitudes toward their first born infants are influenced by the sex of the child, either alone or in combination with other factors. In general, the mothers were very pleased with their infants, whether male or female, although there is a suggestion that if they were disappointed, they were more likely to be displeased with a female infant than with a male. Contrary to what was predicted, whether or not the baby was planned, appeared to be relatively unimportant in the mother's attitude toward her child. A second surprising finding was that the woman's experience of birth was unrelated to her evaluation of her child. The social support system had a significant impact on the mother's evaluation of her child. For both boys and girls, social support from the baby's father was associated with a positive attitude toward infants. Women were significantly more negative toward their infants if they had a poor relationship with the baby's father. Finally, the more acculturated women expressed less positive attitudes toward their newborns; this relationship was slightly stronger for girls than boys.

334. Heer DM ; Falasco D. The socioeconomic status of recent mothers of Mexican origin in Los Angeles County: a comparison of undocumented migrants, legal migrants and native citizens. Paper presented at the Meeting of the Pacific Sociological Association, San Diego, California. April, 1982.

The sampling universe for this study consisted of birth certificates filed in Los Angeles from August 1980 through March 1981. Separate samples were taken for mothers born in and outside the United States. Interviews were conducted in the home about two months after the birth, in Spanish if appropriate. Of births for which one or both parents were reported of **Mexican** or Mexican American origin, it was found that 25% of the mothers were not legally married to the father. The 25% comprised eight percent living in consensual unions, one percent living with a partner not considered to be a spouse, and 16% with no partner present. The overall 25% not legally married in the interview study was almost exactly the same as the inferential estimate of the percent non-married derived from birth certificates for all mothers in California who reported themselves of Mexican or Mexican American origin in 1980. Although there are differences in definition and coverage between study and state estimates, these results do not suggest error in the inferred non-marital birth data for Hispanic mothers.

335. Hoppe SK ; Leon RL. Coping in the barrio: case studies of Mexican American families. **Child Psychiatry Human Development.**

1977 Summer;7(4):264-75.

This paper reports preliminary findings of a study of coping
abilities of **Mexican** American families.   The purpose of the
study was to identify variables related to styles of behavior
that can be characterized as adaptive.   A complex of factors
differentiated families who were judged to be dealing effectively with their environment (copers) from those who were not
(non-copers).   The factors included the health status of the
children, various childrearing attitudes and practices, and
patterns of decision-making as they related to a more general
ability of parents to conceptualize and organize time. Families
that came to be identified as coping were well organized; parents had a clear sense of family history and an expectation for
a future that included realistic goals.   Parents showed affection toward children, and vice versa.   Non-coping parents did
not seem to understand emotional needs or to have a concept of
love and affection.   They displayed little warmth to their
children and stated that it was bad to show affection.

336. *Khalesi MR. Comparison of the parenting attitudes, conflict management styles, and interpersonal behavior patterns of
Anglo, black and Mexican parents.   Doctoral Dissertation, Boul-
der, Colorado, University of Colorado. 1980. DAI;41(8-A):3426.

Parenting and childrearing attitudes,   conflict management
styles, and patterns of interpersonal relations were examined in
questionnaire responses of 184 (of 900 mailed) Anglo, black, and
Mexican American parents.   A significant difference was found
between the attitudes of the Anglo, and black Americans and
those of the Mexican Americans.   A significant interaction between ethnicity and education factors was found, in that positive parenting attitudes were associated with higher levels of
educational attainment for Anglos and blacks, but not for Mexican Americans.   Anglos and Mexican Americans scored higher on
the power approach to conflict than the blacks; Anglos scored
higher than blacks or Chicanos on problem solving approaches to
conflict.   Significant sex effects were found for the adult/
adolescent parenting inventory and the wanted needs for control,
with females scoring higher than males.   Males scored significantly higher than females on power approach to conflict and the
expressed need for control.   The use of power and control in
parenting may increase the probability of child abuse.

337. Leon AM ; Mazur R ; Montalvo E ; Rodriguez M. Self-help
support groups for Hispanic mothers. **Child Welfare.** 1984 May/
Jun;63(3):261-8.

Hispanic families often confront problems raised by the conflicts between Hispanic and Anglo cultural systems and values.
One successful model for assisting Hispanic parents is a self-
help support group based in facilities parents contact within
the regular course of life events.   This approach provides them
with an opportunity to build personal relationships and mutual
support systems with those who share the same interests and
concerns, thereby reducing isolation.   The self-esteem of Hispanic parents can be strengthened by a group approach that
stresses peer problem solving and the development of assertive-
ness, especially in negotiating systems.   This approach provides
them with an opportunity to build mutual support systems, thereby reducing isolation.   The organization and goals of a support
group of this type located in the South Bronx in New York City

are discussed. Replication of the self-help group may be useful
for Hispanic mothers in other communities. Appropriate settings
for initiating these groups are in schools, day care centers,
and Head Start programs.

338. Telles CA. Psychological and physiological adaptation to
pregnancy and childbirth in low income Hispanic women. Doctoral
Dissertation, Boston, Massachusetts, Boston University Graduate
School. 1982. 374 p. DAI;43(4-B):1271.

This study proposed to examine selected social, cultural, personality and endocrinological factors related to the psychological and physiological adaptation to pregnancy and childbirth in
Hispanic women.   One hundred and ten participants were interviewed twice prenatally and twice postpartum. Most psychosocial
variables and premenstrual tension predicted the severity of
pregnancy symptoms, postpartum depression and anxiety and overall psychological adaptation to pregnancy and childbirth.   The
best predictor of more severe postpartum depression, in the
context of other variables, was greater life stress.   Greater
premenstrual tension was the best predictor of more severe
pregnancy symptoms and more difficulty in the overall psychological adaptation. Life stress appeared to exacerbate difficulty
in psychological adaptation and social support appeared to act
as a mediator with a protective function.   The psychosocial
factors and premenstrual tension were not strongly related to
physiological outcome, in terms of maternal or fetal/neonatal
morbidity.   Yet, longer duration of residence in the United
States, and to some extent, a greater level of acculturation
were related to pregnancy, intrapartum and postpartum complications.

339. *U.S. Department of Health and Human Services, National
Center·for Health Statistics. Factors associated with low birth
weight: United States, 1976. By: Taffel S. **Vital and Health
Statistics.** 1980;21(37). 37 p.

This is an analytic study of demographic, socioeconomic, and
health factors associated with low birth weight and a review of
recent trends in low birth rate incidence, based on data reported on birth certificates filed throughout the United States.
Race was found to be one of the more important predictors of
birth weight.   Two factors strongly associated with an infant's
weight at birth are the mother's age at time of birth and the
birth order of the child.   Teenage girls and older mothers are
more likely than are women of other age groups to bear a low
birth weight baby.   Women born in **Puerto Rico** were far more
likely than women born in **Cuba** or **Mexico** to give birth to a low
birth weight baby.   The incidence of low birth weight for infants born to Puerto Rican born mothers was nine percent compared with the very low incidence of five percent for infants
born to mothers born in Cuba and five percent for mothers born
in Mexico.   For almost all racial groups, higher levels of
educational attainment of the mother were associated with a
pronounced decrease in the proportion of low birth weight
babies.

340. *Williams RL ; Binkin NJ ; Clingman EJ. Pregnancy outcomes
among Spanish surnamed women in California. **American Journal of
Public Health** 1986 Apr;76(4):387-91.

The authors compared pregnancy outcomes among United States born and **Mexican** born women having Spanish surnames with U.S. born whites and blacks using California's 1981 matched birth/death cohort file. Maternal risk characteristics between U.S. born black women and U.S. born white women with Spanish surnames were similar. In contrast, Latino women, regardless of national origin, delivered small proportions of low weight infants as compared to blacks. Birth weight specific mortality rates during the fetal and neonatal periods for the offspring of Mexican born Spanish surnamed women were generally higher than those for other ethnic groups. The authors' findings are consistent with the underreporting of postneonatal deaths among Mexican born Latinos, yet suggest that their relatively low reported infant mortality rates compared to blacks can be explained by a more favorable birth weight distribution.

PART FIVE

GENERAL TOPICS

1. Overviews of Hispanics

The papers summarized in this section provide general descriptions of the **number of Hispanics in the United States** and their relative status, as well as some general fertility measures. Specific descriptive variables include **background characteristics, housing characteristics, needs for goods and services,** statistics on the characteristics of **Hispanic families, health services research** on Hispanics, and data on **Hispanic communities,** in particular geographic areas of the U.S.

341. Andrade SJ. **Latino families in the United States: a resource book for family life education.** New York City, Planned Parenthood Federation of America, Education Department. 1983. 79 p.

This resource book assists its readers to acquire facts about Latinos; helps them become aware of the special resources and needs of Latinos; helps them respond appropriately to nuances of Latino behaviors; and helps them become aware of perceptions of Latinos on health care and preventive health practices. This book discusses education, employment, physical security, political participation and representation, and biculturalism. It focuses on **Mexican** Americans, **Puerto Ricans, Cuban** Americans and additional residents of Spanish or Latin American descent. The need to recognize the pluralistic nature of the Latino population with respect to variables such as generations in the United States, racial origin, language practices, religious values, age structure, employment and income differentials, and educational achievement is stressed. Latino family issues, responding to community needs, and the basis for successful Latino family life education are discussed. The cultural and societal sources of stress and support for Latino families interact with each other in a manner that affects the development and promotion of Latino communities. The most significant of these implications relates to the definition of the Latino family. Cultural heritage and identity are major influences on the development of Latinos' self-concepts.

342. Cook AK. Hispanics in the Pacific northwest. Paper presented at the Rural Sociological Society Meetings, Lexington,
Kentucky. August, 1983.

Sources of diversity in the Pacific northwest's Spanish origin
population, up 80% since 1970, was the subject of research based
on 1980 Census data.   Census information for Hispanics (**Mexicans, Puerto Ricans, Cubans**) showed 42% were under 18, compared
to 27% of area whites.   Non-family households were less common
for Hispanics, of whom 56% were married compared to 42% of
whites.   Single women headed 12% of Hispanic families, but only
eight percent of white families.   In the labor force, male
Hispanics had much higher participation rates than white males
in all types of counties.   Contrary to previous findings, Hispanic women also had high participation rates.   Nevertheless,
standard patterns of high Hispanic unemployment prevailed in the
area, as did established patterns of Hispanic education and
poverty levels.   Lower education and higher poverty rates occurred in non-metropolitan and highly agricultural areas for
both Hispanics and whites, but the differences were markedly
greater for Hispanics.   Research is needed in several areas,
including female labor force participation and the processes
which create a disadvantaged population.

343. de la Puente J ; Dillard CD ; Jaramillo P. Health services
research addressing the needs of disadvantaged Hispanics. Paper
presented at the 109th Annual Meeting of the American Public
Health Association. November 4, 1981.

This is a bibliography with abstracts and some tables on the
following topics: 1) research addressing the general Hispanic
population; 2) research on Hispanic elderly; 3) research on
mental health, drug abuse and alcoholism among the Hispanic
population; and 4) research addresssing maternal and child
health care issues.   This synthesis and annotated bibliography
is limited to those studies directed to the underserved Hispanics in the United States.   Probably because the entry of
Hispanics into the professions has been gradual we find a lesser
number of studies conducted by Hispanics. The fields of sociology and mental health appear to be better endowed with results
from Hispanic investigators. Much work has been done addressing
the needs of Hispanics in the southwest, with particular emphasis on maternal and child health.   There appears to be a need
for additional work in health services needed by underserved
Puerto Rican populations residing in the U.S.

344. *Diaz WA. Hispanics: challenges and opportunities. New
York City, Ford Foundation. June, 1984.

In response to the rapid expansion of the Hispanic (**Mexican,
Puerto Rican, Cuban**) population in the United States and its
growing impact on American society, the Ford Foundation's trus-
tees have encouraged the staff to explore whether a new Foundation initiative on the Hispanic population was desirable, and if
so, what form such an initiative might take. The results of the
exploration are presented in this report.   The report first
describes the various groups that comprise the country's Hispanic population, and then examines a number of issues and
challenges facing those groups and the nation as a whole.   After reviewing past and current Foundation efforts to help
address those issues and meet those challenges, the paper presents a new Hispanic focused Foundation program.   The new pro-

gram covers research and policy analysis, efforts to increase Hispanic participation in public affairs, and the need for greater public information and awareness about the Hispanic population among non-Hispanics.

345. Fitzpatrick JP ; Parker LT. Hispanic Americans in the eastern United States. In: Gordon MM, ed. **America as a multicultural society.** 1981;454:98-110.

The eastern part of the United States contains a large and growing Hispanic minority. If present trends continue, all Hispanics will constitute the largest minority in the U.S. by the year 2000. Their influence is already felt in the social and political life of the nation. The largest concentration of Hispanics, mainly **Puerto Ricans,** in the east is found in the New York City area. **Cubans** predominate in the Dade County area of Florida, with large numbers also in New York City and in the northern New Jersey area. Newcomers from **Santo Domingo, Central America** and **South America** are found in the New York City and other large eastern cities. These populations vary in age, color, education, and occupation. Cubans, Central Americans and South Americans tend to be at the level of the American middle class; Puerto Ricans and Dominicans tend to be at lower socioeconomic levels. Puerto Ricans are steadily progressing in New York City in terms of political representation and organizational activity. Hispanics may play as important a role in the U.S. during the next century as Americans from European backgrounds have played in the present century.

346. Gurak DT. Dominican migrants in New York. Paper prepared for the Hispanic Research Center, Bronx, New York, Fordham University. (Unpublished) 1983. 7 p.

Selected socioeconomic and demographic characteristics of both **Dominican** and **Colombian** migrants according to sex are displayed. Demographic characteristics include age at arrival and average United States duration. Socioeconomic factors include level of education, percent in the labor force and total household size. The main reasons for moving to the U.S. are rejoining family members, and looking for work or improving one's economic situation. A chart showing relationships with relatives at various stages of the migration process is included as well as selected measures of assistance to relatives. The likely source of assistance (relatives in the U.S., relatives in one's home country, one's employer, U.S. government agencies, or a bank or financial institution) in a financial crisis is also reported according to sex, ethnicity and duration in the U.S. Finally, determinants of indicators of assimilation are shown. Such determinants are ethnicity, sex, education, years in the U.S., being in the labor force prior to migration, household income, currently married, and percent of types of aid received from relatives at immigration.

347. Klitz SI. Cross-cultural communication: the Hispanic community of Connecticut. A human services staff development training manual, Research in Education. 1980. 65 p.

This manual was designed for use by Title XX field training personnel involved in providing services for **Puerto Ricans** in Connecticut. The manual is intended to develop cross-cultural awareness by introducing the reader to the cultural orientations, social systems and values of Puerto Ricans and other

Hispanics.   Included are background information on Puerto Rican
geography, history, economy, and politics; a description of
Hispanic value systems, family structure, religion, courtship,
marriage practices, and health practices; a discussion of the
Puerto Rican experience in the United States in politics, housing, employment and education; and a community social and health
service model for Puerto Ricans.   Also included are sample
lessons for a Spanish language curriculum and a directory of
Spanish speaking resource organizations in Connecticut.

348.   Massey DS. Dimensions of the new immigration to the United
States and the prospects for assimilation. **Annual Review of
Sociology.** 1981;7:57-85.

This paper provides an overview of the substantial increase in
migration to the United States that has occurred over the past
two decades.   The author draws on research from a variety of
disciplines in order to describe who these immigrants are (including **Mexicans, Puerto Ricans, Cubans, Central Americans** and
South Americans) and how they are faring.   He covers both legal
and illegal immigration and presents estimates of a total of
eight million immigrants (excluding Puerto Ricans) for the decade of the 1970s.   Various characteristics of migrants are
discussed, including family behavior, fertility, residential
segregation, intermarriage, and social mobility.

349.   Momeni JA. **Demography of racial and ethnic minorities in
the United States: an annotated bibliography with a review
essay.** Westport, Connecticut/London, England, Greenwood Press.
1984. 292 p.

An annotated bibliography on the demography of racial and ethnic
minorities in the United States is presented.   The bibliography
is organized by seven major topics and within those topics
alphabetically by author.   These topics are minority group status and fertility patterns; minority nuptiality, family, and
fertility outside marriage; fertility regulation and minorities;
minority health and mortality; minority migration, urbanization,
and ecology; minority status, economy, and demography; and
minority population growth, composition, distribution, and vital
rates. The bibliography deals with various racial and ethnic
minorities: American Indians, Asians and Pacific Islanders,
Hispanics (**Mexicans, Puerto Ricans, Cubans**), and the Jewish
population of the U.S.   A general review of the demography of
racial and ethnic minorities in the U.S. is also presented from
a political and sociodemographic perspective.   An author index
and an index of minority groups and subjects are included.

350.   *National Council of La Raza. Socioeconomic demographic
highlights of Hispanic Americans. Washington, D.C. 1982. 22 p.

Key socioeconomic and demographic characteristics of Hispanic
Americans are summarized in narrative fashion in the first part
of this report, while the second part contains charts and
graphs.   Hispanic subgroups dealt with are Latin Americans,
Cubans, Mexican Americans, and **Puerto Ricans**. Subjects covered
include their percentage in the total United States population,
racial identity, population distribution, location of school age
population, years of schooling, occupational distribution, unemployment, income, age, household size, and place of birth.

351.   *New York City Department of City Planning. The Puerto

Rican New Yorkers: a recent history of their distribution and population and household characteristics. By: Mann E et al. December, 1982.

Section I of this report begins by discussing the **Puerto Rican** population in the context of the growth and distribution of the total population of Spanish/Hispanic origin or descent. Changes in this relationship between 1970 and 1980 are presented. The redistribution of the Puerto Rican population in the United States during the last decade is shown in table form and discussed briefly. Finally, the spatial redistribution of the Puerto Rican population within New York City by borough and community since 1950 is examined. Section II presents full count 1980 Census data for the City and for the Puerto Rican population. Nineteen pairs of tables of demographic and housing characteristics are included, contrasting and comparing the Puerto Rican population and housing characteristics with those of the City as a whole. Section III, presenting 1970 and 1980 full count subject matter for the City wide Puerto Rican population and housing units, contains ten tables and analyses. The tables were designed to maximize the only information from the 1970 Census which is comparable to that of 1980. It is noted that all Census data in this report must be considered preliminary pending the outcome of litigation over a possible population undercount.

352. U.S. Department of Commerce, Bureau of the Census. **Condition of Hispanics in America today.** U.S. Government Printing Office. 1983.

This report was originally prepared as testimony before the House Subcommittee on Census and Population in September, 1983. Data were extracted from the wealth of statistics on the Hispanic population gathered from censuses and current surveys. This document presents a statistical overview of the current conditions of Hispanics (**Mexicans, Puerto Ricans, Cubans**) as well as major demographic changes during the last decade. Included are statistics on population growth and fertility levels.

353. *U.S. Department of Health and Human Services, National Center for Health Services Research. **Hispanic health services research.** Research Proceedings Series. September, 1980. (DHHS Publication No.80-3288).

This report contains the proceedings of the first Hispanic Health Services Research Conference, which was supported by a grant from the National Center for Health Services Research with additional funding from the Veterans Administration. The conference addressed the health problems of Hispanic populations in the United States, identified needed areas of research, and recommended methodologies appropriate for conducting health research among Hispanic populations. The recommendations of the conference are presented in the individual reports of the four task forces, which focused on the impact of national, regional, state and local health policies on health services for Hispanics; sociocultural influences and health services delivery for Hispanics; resource development strategies for conducting health services research among Hispanic populations; and facilitation of the timely dissemination and assessment of Hispanic health services research.

354. U.S. Department of Health and Human Services, National

Center for Health Services Research. Hispanic health services research: a preliminary bibliography. Research Report Series. April, 1981.

This bibliography includes research on the financing, delivery and organization of health services for Hispanics. It is an accumulation of papers, primarily unpublished, prepared by authors at the National Center for Health Services Research and elsewhere. A listing of reports prepared for the first Hispanic Health Services Research Conference is included.

355. *Zambrana RE. Work, family, and health: Latina women in transition. Bronx, New York, Fordham University. Hispanic Research Center. 1982. 19 p.

The ten papers in this monograph examine the background, characteristics, social roles, and social/psychological needs of Hispanic women in the United States (especially **Mexicans, Puerto Ricans, Cubans** in New York City). Based on recent research and other studies, the articles focus on: 1) the interplay between sociocultural factors and Puerto Rican women's mental health needs; 2) the influence of the women's movement on the self-concepts and social roles of Puerto Rican women of different generations; 3) problems related to changing family roles, isolation, ethnic identity, acculturation and help seeking among Hispanic women in suburban New York; 4) clinical findings concerning sex roles and acculturation among Puerto Rican adolescents; 5) relationships between cultural attitudes toward mental illness and use of community mental health services among Puerto Rican women; 6) voluntary reproductive sterilization among Hispanic women in a Connecticut community; 7) determinants of Hispanic children's health status and use of health facilities; 8) patterns and determinants of women's labor force participation in Puerto Rico from 1899 to 1975; 9) the demography, economic profiles, and changing roles and status of Cuban women; and 10) influences of economic factors, Hispanic culture, and stereotypes on Hispanic women's family roles.

2. Hispanic Males

Although studies which include data on such topics as adolescent fatherhood and contraceptive method choice by Hispanic males might most correctly fall into the respective categories for fertility and contraceptive use, they have been organized into a separate category because of the scarcity of male data and because of particular interest on the part of many researchers and health program personnel. A few studies of high school students have included questions on sexuality and contraceptive use by Hispanic males. Some statistics also come from the National Longitudinal Survey of Youth, although the authors note that the NLS fertility data for males are less reliable than the data for females.

356. *Boria-Berna MC ; Gordon M. The role of male counselors in a family planning service. In: Sobrero AJ and Harvey RM, eds. **Advances in planned parenthood, Vol. 7.** Princeton, Excerpta Medica. 1972. p. 69-78.

Questionnaires were administered to 128 puerperal women in the Metropolitan Hospital Center in New York, and to their male partners. Demographic data were obtained as well as attitudes toward pregnancy and birth control. Women were asked questions concerning what they perceived to be their male partner's attitude toward the same topics. There was a discrepancy of 54% between the man's supposed attitude toward future pregnancies and his real attitude among **Puerto Rican** couples; the inconsistencies were 33% for blacks and 40% for whites. Latin women were more conditioned than other groups to accept their partner's decision to use or not to use contraception. Some 55% of the men interviewed did not like contraceptives, but reluctantly agreed to accept it; only 34% said they liked birth control. Seventy percent of the men, however, indicated they would like to learn more about birth control. It is, therefore, considered important to have male counselors available in family planning programs. Two male counselors at the Metropolitan Hospital Center contacted about 550 men within five months and found 87% of the cases receptive.

357. *Feigenbaum E. Males and family planning: an attitudinal survey of 1,200 teen and adult males in Merced County. Merced County, California, Merced County Health Department, Health Status Survey. (Unpublished) 1978. 34 p.

This is a report on a study of two groups of males in Merced County, California to determine their attitudes toward the male's role in family planning. Three hundred and five teenage males and 903 adult males were interviewed, with an attempt to reflect the percentages of various ethnic groups in the County (made up of white Americans, **Mexican** Americans, Mexicans and black Americans). The teenagers and adult males were asked basically the same questions, the difference being that the teenagers' questions were weighted toward the hypothetical while the adults' were more experiential. The main point of the survey was to discover the following: 1) attitude toward sex education in schools; 2) attitude toward birth control; 3) feelings about contraception for teens; 4) desire to be a teen-age father; 5) whether male, female or both have responsibility for birth control; 6) where family planning should be taught; 7) who would use contraception; 8) where would they prefer to receive family planning information; 9) awareness of available family planning services; 10) how many had been to county family planning clinics; 11) knowledge of male and female contraceptive devices; and 12) knowledge of vasectomy.

358. *Finkel ML. Male adolescent sexual behavior: policy impli-cations. Paper presented at the Annual Meeting of the American Public Health Association, New Orleans, Louisiana. October, 1974. 29 p.

It is the intent of this study to begin to place the male adolescent in his proper perspective and to examine his behavior ana attitudes toward human sexuality. A total of 421 male adolescents comprising three sociocultural groups (black, His-panic, and white) were given a questionnaire to complete. The males were students at three lower/middle income high schools in the northeast. Eighty-four percent of the black males and 75% of the Hispanic males had had sexual intercourse as compared to 48% of the white males. Black and Hispanic males also had their first coital experience at the earliest ages; mean age at first coitus for black males was 11.6 years; and the mean age at first coitus for Hispanic males was 13 years. The white males began their coital activity at a much later age; mean age was 14.5 years. Black and Hispanic males relied on withdrawal or the douche, while the white males relied on the condom to prevent pregnancies at last coitus. Black and Hispanic males reported using similar birth control methods at last coitus as 32% of the black males and 32% of the Hispanic males reported using with-drawal or the douche at last coitus. One-fourth (26%) of the black males and 25% of the Hispanic males used no birth control at last coitus.

359. *Finkel ML. Policy decisions and research on adolescent sexual behavior. Doctoral Dissertation, New York City, New York University. 1980. 191 p. DAI;41(12-B):4472.

Government policies and empirical studies concerning adolescent sexuality were reviewed as background to a study of adolescent males' sexual knowledge, attitudes, and practice. Government policy has shifted from one of benign neglect to one of substan-tial financial and administrative involvement. However, the

focus is on the pregnant female.   It is contended that current
policies are narrowly defined, limited in scope, and not respon-
sive to adolescents' needs.   Few programs are designed to
include   the teenage male and relatively little is   known   about
his sexual behavior.   Findings show that 69% of the 421 male
high school students surveyed were sexually experienced; half
began sexual activity before the age of 14.   At last coitus, 55%
used   no contraceptives or relied on ineffective methods.   Differences in sexual activity and contraceptive use were   evident
among   black,   Hispanic,   and white males and among age groups
within   each of the sociocultural categories.   Results indicate
that the respondents were most informed about male birth control
devices,   fairly knowledgeable about female contraceptives, and
least knowledgeable about the female menstrual cycle.   Recommendations are made for improved present policies toward adolescent
sexuality.

360. *Finkel ML ; Finkel DJ. Male adolescent contraceptive
utilization. **Adolescence.** 1978 Fall;13(51):443-51.

Four hundred and twenty-one male students enrolled in three high
schools in a large, northeastern city completed a 46 item questionnaire in the spring of 1974 in order to examine contraceptive utilization among a sample of sexually active, urban high
school males.   Thirty-four percent of the sample are black; 38%
are Hispanic (**Puerto Rican, Cuban, Dominican, Haitian**); and 32%
are white.   Those who reported using the condom and those whose
female partners used birth control are classified as being
effective contraceptors.   Fifty-five percent of the sample are
ineffective contraceptors.   The findings indicate almost identi-
cal percentages for black and Hispanic males as effective and
ineffective contraceptors, but the majority of white males (59%)
are effective contraceptors.   Two-thirds (68%) of those 15 years
and younger are ineffective contraceptors while 63% of those 18
and 19 years old are effective contraceptors.   Those 16 and 17
years old are fairly evenly divided between effective and ineffective contraceptors.   White males are more consistent in their
use of the condom than their black and Hispanic counterparts.
The most frequent reasons for failing to use contraceptives
demonstrate   that the males in this sample either were not prepared for sexual intercourse or were not concerned if their
partner became pregnant.

361. *Finkel ML ; Finkel DJ. Sexual and contraceptive knowledge,   attitudes and behavior of male adolescents. **Family Planning Perspectives.** 1975 Nov/Dec;7(6):256-60.

A 1974 profile of male adolescent sexuality and contraceptive
knowledge is based on a survey of 421 students, aged 12 to 19,
from three urban high schools in a northeastern American city.
Thirty percent of the respondents were black, 38% Hispanic
(**Puerto Rican, Cuban, Dominican, Haitian**), and 32% white; mean
age was 16.3.   Male friends proved to be the most frequent
source of sexual and contraceptive knowledge; less than 11% of
the boys within each ethnic group had acquired information from
a family member.   A majority of the respondents understood the
condom's contraceptive use but far fewer were aware of the
protection it offers against venereal disease.   Two-thirds were
aware of the contraceptive unreliability of the douche, but only
about one-third knew that pregnancy could result from the practice of withdrawal during coitus.   While two-thirds knew of
sperm's survival time after ejaculation, less than half could

identify the conception phase of the menstrual cycle.   Mean age
for initial sexual experience was 12.8 years; subsequent sexual
activity appeared sporadic.   At last coitus, 55% of the sexually
active respondents used no contraception, or relied on withdrawal or their partner's douching.   Among all sexually active
males,   only 15% reported using a condom for each coitus, while
50% reported hardly ever or never using one.

362. *Johnson LB ; Staples RE. Family planning and the young
minority male: a pilot project. **Family Coordinator.** 1979
Oct;28(4):535-43.

In Los Angeles the first coordinated program, the Young Inner-
City Males Project, sought to reach black, Spanish speaking,
Asian,   and American Indian males in relation to family life
education, family planning, and parental responsibilities. Race
and cultural practices are two significant factors which influence the perception of sex roles and sexuality.   In the Latino
community,   it is important to recognize the impact of significant others.   These two groups are known to have strong con-
sanguine and fictive kinship ties which serve as emotional,
psychological, and financial support systems.   The right and
obligations of non-consanguine compadrazgo (godparents), are
similar to any blood relative and are highly valued in the
Mexican American community.   The role of the male virility cult
and family planning in the Chicano and black community is still
another illustration.   Within these cultures there is evidence
that a link exists between the ability to have sexual relations
with women, the subsequent birth of children, and the self-image
of the male.   We cannot overlook the link between economic
opportunities and the young minority male's attitudes toward and
enactment of the father role.

363. Laguna JN. The Puerto Rican adolescent father: a psychological perspective. Doctoral Dissertation, New York City, City
University of New York. April, 1984. 127 p. DAI;44(10-B):3200.

Thirty **Puerto Rican** adolescent males from the New York metropolitan area were interviewed about their attitudes and behavior
on the variables of family, ethnicity, intimacy, and fatherhood.
Two groups were compared: 15 unwed fathers, and 15 unwed non-
fathers.   Ethnicity was supported on the hypothesis that fathers
affiliated more closely with Puerto Rican peers than non-fathers
(Fisher Exact Probability Test, p<.05).   A reanalysis showed
significant differences in attitude, with non-fathers having
more positive attitudes concerning Puerto Rican ethnocultural
membership than fathers (Fisher Exact Probability Test, p<.05).
The second hypothesis positing differences between the groups in
their designation as Puerto Rican was not supported. Fatherhood
was not supported on: 1) that fathers and non-fathers differed
in their real perceptions of fatherhood; 2) that the two groups
differed on the role modeling of their own fathers; 3) that
there would be differences concerning the Puerto Rican father as
being different from fathers in other groups; and 4) that more
fathers than non-fathers would be sons of unwed fathers.

364. Zinn MB. Chicano men and masculinity. **Journal of Ethnic
Studies.** 1982 Summer;10(2):29-44.

The assumption that male dominance among Chicanos (**Mexicans**) is
exclusively a cultural phenomenon is contradicted by much evidence.   The author raises the point that further understanding

of larger societal conditions in which masculinity is embedded and expressed is needed. A disturbing relationship exists among race, sex, and class; to the extent that social inequality limits men's access to resources, it also contributes to sexual stratification. To the extent that systems of social inequality limit men's access to societally valued resources, they also contribute to sexual stratification. Men in some social categories will continue to draw upon and accentuate their masculinity as a socially valued resource. This in turn poses serious threats to sexual equality. We are compelled to move the study of masculinity beyond narrow confines of subcultural roles, and to make the necessary theoretical and empirical connections between the contingencies of sex and gender and the social order.

Author Index

Abney GA, 132
Abrahamse AF, 1
Abramson PR, 51
Aguirre BE, 131
Alba F, 195
Alcalay R, 52-53
Alex PL, 324
Almaguer T, 165
Alvarez A, 101
Alvirez D, 54, 196
Amaro HD, 55
Andrade SJ, 56-58, 267-268, 341
Angel R, 160
Arce CH, 132
Archdiocese of New York, 180
Atkinson DR, 232
Auerbach S, 170
Aviaro H, 181

Bacharach CA, 169, 279, 284
Bachu A, 197
Backstrand J, 300
Barnett C, 101
Barrera V, 300
Barron E, 295
Bassoff BZ, 59
Bauman KE, 261
Bean FD, 2-12, 32, 60, 65, 130, 139-143, 145, 196, 198-201, 331
Becerra RM, 13, 61, 79, 272
Beckman LJ, 14
Benedicto M, 170
Bennet CF, 269
Berkman-Sherry L, 305
Binkin NJ, 340
Bird HR, 62
Blaschke TJ, 310

Bloom B, 254, 264
Bonta D, 233
Boria-Berna MC, 356
Borrero M, 300
Borup JH, 63
Borus ME, 64
Boswell TD, 204
Boulette TR, 332
Bradshaw BS, 198, 200-201
Bragonier JR, 182
Bristow C, 171
Brown SV, 306
Browning HL, 27, 145

Cadena MA, 172
Caetano DF, 71
Caldiz L, 53
Camarillo A, 165
Cameron O, 239
Canino G, 62
Cannon-Bonventre K, 307
Cardenas G, 46
Carmichael JS, 30, 93, 278
Cazares RB, 133, 155
Charnowski KM, 166
Cherlin A, 134
Chow W, 92
Chung HC, 308
Clingman EJ, 340
Cochrane SH, 65
Cohn MR, 171
Collins M, 158
Cook AK, 342
Cooney RS, 15, 66, 135-136, 157, 318
Cressy MK, 234
Cromwell RE, 67
Crowley JE, 64
Cullen RM, 4, 204

Cummings M, 270
Cummings S, 270
Curry JP, 16
Curtis RL Jr, 60
Cypress B, 258

Daily EF, 296
Darabi KF, 68, 202, 248, 320
Darrow WW, 167
Davis C, 203
Davis SM, 69-70
De Anda D, 13
Decker DL, 71
de la Puente J, 343
Diaz WA, 344
Dillard CD, 343
Doyle MB, 173

Eberstein IW, 137, 139-140
Eckard E, 255, 265
Edington A, 246
Edington E, 72
Eisen M, 73-74, 92
Engle PL, 333
Erhardt CL, 184
Erickson PI, 75
Esparza R, 76
Ezzati I, 271

Falasco D, 17, 334
Falk WW, 77
Falkowski CK, 77
Family Planning Council of
  New York City, 235
Fan MYC, 18
Farrell J, 138
Farris BE, 78
Feigenbaum E, 357
Fielder EP, 61, 79, 272
Finkel DJ, 360-361
Finkel ML, 358-361
Fischer NA, 19
Fisher-Burton N, 183
Fitzpatrick JP, 148, 345
Fletcher PL, 80
Ford K, 20, 227
Forrest JD, 249
Foster JE, 255, 257
Friedman JS, 275, 285
Frisbie WP, 5, 133, 137, 139-
  147, 156

Gant LM, 110
Garcia Coll CT, 309
Garcia-Nunez J, 288-289, 293
Gibbs CE, 273
Gillespie DG, 243
Glenn ND, 78

Gold EM, 184
Golden JS, 168
Golden M, 168
Goldscheider C, 21
Gonzalez A, 81
Gordon M, 356
Graham EH, 320-321
Gray SS, 82-83
Green V, 91
Grinker WJ, 313
Guarnaccia P, 300
Gurak DT, 22-23, 37, 148-149,
  319, 346
Gurel L, 30, 93, 278
Gutierrez M, 273

Haggstrom GW, 310-311
Halberstein RA, 24
Hansen GL, 77
Hanson RA, 84
Harris D, 185, 188
Harris MB, 69-70
Harvey SM, 274
Haub C, 203
Hawkes GR, 85
Hays L, 72
Heath LL, 25, 108
Heer DM, 17, 334
Heinrich A, 168
Held L, 312
Heller PL, 87
Hendershot GE, 207, 260-261
Henry M, 123
Hnat SA, 110
Hoffman LW, 86
Holck SE, 275-276, 285, 304
Holland A, 232
Holmes KA, 129
Hoppe SK, 87, 152, 335
Horn MC, 169, 262, 284
Horowitz R, 88
Hotvedt ME, 89
Hough RL, 124
Howell VV, 327
Huling T, 171
Hunter K, 297
Hurrel RM, 66

Inman JM, 143

Jacobziner H, 184
Jaffe AJ, 204
Jaramillo P, 343
Johnson CA, 26
Johnson D, 126
Johnson LB, 362
Jones JE, 236, 240-241, 244-
  245

Jones V, 268
Juarez RZ, 205

Kahn JR, 307, 322-323
Kalmuss D, 241
Kanouse DE, 310
Kaplan CP, 75, 233
Kaplan HB, 38
Kaufman R, 141-142
Kaye JW, 281
Kazen PM, 27
Kearl MC, 150
Keefe SE, 151
Kelly WR, 145, 147
Khalesi MR, 336
King AG, 331
King CD, 25, 108
Klitenick P, 93, 278
Klitz SI, 90, 347
Kramer MJ, 186
Kranau EJ, 91
Kritz MM, 149
Krivo LJ, 145
Krubiner P, 28
Kunkes CH, 281
Kurtines W, 47

Laguna JN, 363
Lee ES, 29, 39
Leibowitz A, 92
Lennhoff S, 120
Leon AM, 337
Leon RL, 335
Levy SB, 313
Lewit S, 194
Lindemann C, 277
Linn MW, 30, 93, 278, 297
Linsley TF, 9
Lisowski W, 310
Looper T, 238
Lopez DE, 31, 40
Lowe EW, 182

Macisco JJ Jr, 37
Manis JD, 86
Mann ES, 206, 351
Marcum JP, 6, 10-11, 19, 32,
    60
Marin BV, 94, 237
Marin G, 94, 237
Markides KS, 138, 152
Marsiglio W, 317
Martin HW, 273
Martin SS, 38
Martinez AL, 314
Martinez-Manautou J, 293
Massey DS, 348
Mazur R, 337
McCall PL, 144

McCarthy J, 134
Meadow A, 120
Michael RT, 33
Miller MV, 95
Min K, 136
Mindel CH, 153
Minkler D, 238
Mirande A, 96-97, 117
Mitchell JO, 98
Mittlebach FG, 154
Moerk E, 99
Momeni JA, 349
Montalvo E, 337
Montes JM, 100
Mookherjee HN, 34
Moore JW, 154
Morgenthau JE, 192, 239
Moriuchi KD, 51
Morris L, 276
Morris R, 324
Morrison PA, 1, 310-311
Mosena PW, 315
Mosher WD, 176, 207, 262, 279,
    284
Mosher, WP, 292
Moss N, 101, 174
Mott FL, 35-36, 102-103, 208-
    209, 316-317
Mott SH, 102-103
Mumford SD, 298
Murguia E, 133, 150, 155-156
Murillo-Rhode I, 104
Mutchler J, 141, 144-145

Namerow PB, 68, 105, 236, 240-
    242, 245, 281
Nathan B, 170
National Council of La Raza,
    350
Nelson FG, 184-185, 188-191
Nelson VE, 158
New York City Dept. of Plan-
    ning, 351
New York City Dept. of Health,
    Bureau of Health Statistics
    and Analysis, 210
Nicholas N, 296
Nies CM, 280
Notzon F, 263

O'Connell M, 211, 219
O'Hare D, 170, 185, 191
Okada LM, 243
Okada Y, 42, 213
Opitz W, 46, 146-147, 199
Ortiz CG, 187
Ortiz ET, 59,
Ortiz V, 66, 202, 318-319
Owings JA, 326

Padilla AM, 94, 237
Pakter J, 185, 188-191
Parker LT, 345
Pasquariella B, 301-302
Perlman J, 271
Perry LB, 51
Petchesky RP, 299
Philliber SG, 68, 105, 236, 242, 244-245, 247, 281, 320-321
Pippin MU, 106
Polgar S, 282
Poliak J, 192
Polit DF, 322-323
Pomeroy R, 283
Poston DL, 142-143, 145
Powers MG, 37
Pratt WF, 284
Price S, 168

Ralph N, 246
Ramirez M 3rd, 107
Rao PS, 239
Rawlings SW, 162
Richardson JA, 295
Rindfuss RR, 212
Ritchey S, 324
Robbins C, 38
Roberts RE, 29, 39
Rochat RW, 275-276, 285, 289, 293-294, 304
Rodriquez M, 337
Rogeness GA, 324
Rogers CC, 211
Rogler LH, 15, 66, 157
Romero A, 124
Roper BS, 25, 108
Rosenhouse-Persson S, 109
Rothenberg PB, 247, 325
Rothman J, 110
Rothstein F, 282
Rudov MH, 252
Ruiz RA, 67
Rumberger RW, 64
Russell Briefel R, 271

Sabagh G, 31, 40, 109, 111, 286
Salazar D, 112
Salazar SA, 175
Salvo JJ, 206
Sanchez RB, 113
Santa Clara County Health Dept., 114
Santangelo N, 252
Santos R, 64
Satterfiled D, 120
Schensul SL, 300
Schoen R, 41, 158
Schroder E, 15

Schwartz DB, 248
Scopetta MA, 47
Scott CS, 287
Scott W, 277
Scrimshaw SC, 301-302, 333
Scrimshaw SM, 75
Scriven GD, 16
Shane R, 278
Shapiro D, 64
Sibirsky S, 308
Singh S, 290
Slesinger DP, 42, 213
Smidt R, 333
Smith JC, 275, 285, 288-289, 293-294, 304
Soloway RD, 171
Sorenson AM, 43-44, 115
Sparer G, 303
Spencer G, 214
Staples RE, 116-117, 362
Staton RD, 118
Stein SR, 297
Steinhoff PG, 193
Stephen EH, 4, 46, 199
Svigir M, 191
Sweet JA, 159, 215-216
Swicegood CG, 4, 7-11, 45-46, 331
Szapocznik J, 47

Taffel SM, 177, 225, 339
Takai RT, 326
Tamez EG, 119
Tanfer K, 37
Tannen MB, 323
Taylor M, 85
Teberg AJ, 327
Telles CA, 338
Testa M, 328
Tharp RG, 120
Thorton JC, 239
Tienda M, 48, 121, 160
Tietze C, 194
Tittle CK, 122
Torres A, 217-218, 249, 283, 290
Torres MG, 58
Trevino MC, 172
Tuma NB, 33
Tyrer LB, 219

Udry JR, 250
Uhlenberg PR, 21, 49, 161
US Dept. of Commerce, Bureau of the Census, 162-163, 220-222, 352
US Dept. of Commerce, National Technical Information Services, 251

US DHHS, Centers for Disease
    Control, 223-224, 291
US DHHS, Health Resources
    Administration, 252
US DHHS, National Center for
    Health Services Research,
    353-354
US DHHS, National Center for
    Health Statistics, 169, 176,
    225-227, 253-265, 292, 339
Urdaneta ML, 266

Valdez A, 164-165
Valencia-Weber G, 91
Varga PE, 325
Vaughan D, 303
Veatch RM, 123
Vega WA, 124
Ventura SJ, 177, 226, 228

Waite LJ, 1
Waite MS, 51
Waltman NM, 233
Warren CW, 50, 275-276, 285,
    288-289, 293-294, 304
Warwick DP, 125
Waterman C, 126
Webb N, 93
Weed P, 30
Weisbord RG, 127
Weller RH, 37
Welti VS, 329
Westoff CF, 229
Whiteford LM, 230
Widhalm MV, 173
Willette J, 203
Williams D, 196
Williams JE, 128-129
Williams RL, 340
Williamson N, 125
Wingert WA, 327
Winzelberg A, 232
Wittenberg CK, 178
Wood CH, 12, 130

Young WR III, 330

Zambrana RE, 355
Zellman GL, 73-74
Zinn MB, 364
Zuelzer M, 324

Subject Index

Abortion, 28, 50, 55, 68, 73,
92-93, 109, 123, 179-194,
208-210, 219, 235, 278, 281,
296, 314

Academic ability, 1

Acculturation and assimilation, 4-5, 9, 11, 13, 15,
22-23, 29, 42-43, 45-47, 79,
91, 116, 118, 120-121, 165,
213, 272, 277, 348, 355

Adolescent pregnancy and
childbearing, 28, 38, 113,
171, 173-175, 187, 305-330

Adolescents, 1, 10, 13-14, 26,
28, 33, 35-39, 42-44, 49,
51, 58-59, 61, 63-64, 68-74,
79-81, 92, 97, 99-103, 105-
107, 109, 111-115, 118-119,
122, 134, 136, 140, 142,
146, 153, 159, 162-163, 166,
168, 170-171, 173-176, 178,
182, 184-194, 199-201, 205,
207-210, 212-213, 216-220,
223-224, 226, 228, 231, 233-
236, 239-249, 252-255, 257-
265, 267, 270-277, 281, 283-
286, 288-294, 302-303, 305-
324, 326-330, 333, 336, 339-
340, 344, 350-351, 353, 355-
363

Attitudes:
alienation, 87
authoritarianism, 96, 107
familism, 27, 60, 78, 82-84,
87-88, 95-96, 107, 110,

familism (cont'd)
117-119, 121, 124, 126
fatalism, 38, 67, 78
machismo, 27, 67, 88, 90,
96-97, 104, 117-119, 125-
126, 266, 270, 298
religiosity, 35, 40, 54, 67,
286
self-esteem, 38, 119, 312
sex-related, 51-130, 180,
198, 287
sex roles, 14, 35, 55, 60,
80-81, 85, 90-91, 95, 97,
102-103, 112, 120, 128,
270, 355
traditionalism, 108

Attitudes toward:
abortion, 55, 68, 93, 109,
180-181, 183, 187, 278,
281, 314
childlessness, 76
children, 76, 86, 92, 100,
122
contraceptive use, 13, 55,
61, 68, 88-89, 93-94, 98,
100, 114, 268, 278, 281,
286-287, 302, 357
gender preference, 130
marriage, 58-60, 84, 89, 90,
122
population policy, 123, 125,
127
pregnancy and childbearing,
13, 55, 92-93, 100-101,
113, 170-178, 270, 294,
304, 363
rape, 128-129
sex education, 51, 68, 105,
357

sexual activity, 55, 61, 63,
    68, 93, 113, 313-314
sterilization, 125

Bolivian, 91

Central and South American,
    127, 148, 160, 177, 204,
    217, 222, 226, 345, 348

Chicano (see Mexican)

Childlessness, 76, 214

Colombian 149, 206, 346

Communication:
    husband/wife, 66, 282
    parent/child, 51, 277

Contraceptive use, 13, 35, 42,
    50, 55, 61, 68, 74, 88-89,
    93-94, 99-100, 114, 166,
    179, 200, 209, 217-219, 224,
    230, 234, 239-245, 247-248,
    253-257, 259-262, 264-265,
    267-294, 302, 357-358, 360

Counseling and counselors, 53,
    232, 244, 295, 356

Cuban, 6, 20, 23, 30, 36, 47,
    52, 58, 91, 93, 113, 131,
    142-145, 148, 177, 197, 203-
    204, 210, 217-219, 222, 225,
    228, 240, 251, 278, 287,
    331, 339, 341-342, 344-345,
    348-350, 352, 355, 360-361

Decision-making, 66, 85, 183,
    187

Dominican, 37, 148-149, 206,
    248, 345-346, 360-361

Extended family, 52, 116, 124,
    151, 153, 165, 314, 346

Familism (see Attitudes,
familism)

Family characteristics, 1, 33,
    36-37

Family planning clinics, 224,
    231-294, 356

Family size desires, expecta-
    tions, preferences, 3, 14,
    30, 43-44, 48-49, 54, 64-
    65, 72, 75, 93-94, 99,
    102-103, 111, 115, 200,

Family size desires (cont'd)
    208, 220, 237, 286

Fertility, general conse-
quences of:
    education, 7, 9-11, 18-19,
        26, 35, 37, 39, 45, 50,
        109, 195, 208, 215, 307,
        310, 312, 318-319, 323,
        326, 328, 330
    labor force participation,
        11, 26, 37, 77, 196, 206,
        308, 319, 323, 328, 331
    low birth weight, 177, 210,
        226, 339-340
    parenting skills and styles,
        305-330, 333, 335-336
    psychological consequences,
        309, 312, 320, 338
    subsequent fertility, 308,
        316, 322, 328

Fertility, general determinants of:
    academic ability, 1
    acculturation and assimila-
        tion, 4-5, 9, 11, 13, 15,
        21-23, 29, 42-43, 45-47,
        79, 91, 116, 118, 120-121,
        165, 213, 272, 277, 348,
        355
    education, 7, 9-11, 18-19,
        26, 35, 37, 39, 45, 50,
        109, 195, 207, 214, 307,
        310, 312, 318-319, 323,
        326, 328, 330
    family characteristics, 1,
        33, 36-37
    family size desires, expec-
        tations, preferences, 3,
        14, 30, 43-44, 48-49, 54,
        64-65, 72, 75, 93-94, 99,
        102-103, 111, 115, 200,
        208, 220, 237, 286
    gender preference, 130
    generation, 4, 7-9, 11, 15,
        32, 45, 49, 202, 237
    income, 2-3, 11-12, 17-18,
        39, 215
    labor force participation,
        11, 26, 37, 77, 196, 206,
        308, 319, 323, 328, 331
    legal status, 17
    migration, 212-213, 230
    minority group status, 2-3,
        5-8, 10, 15, 18-19, 21-
        23, 31-32, 34, 39, 41, 48,
        50, 207
    religion, 44, 54
    religiosity, 35, 40, 54, 67,
        286
    socioeconomic status, 1-3,

socioeconomic status
(cont'd)
   7-9, 11-12, 17-19, 21-23,
   28-29, 31-32, 34, 38-41,
   48-50, 198, 202, 206, 216
urbanization, 24, 196

Machismo (see Attitudes,
machismo)

Males, 67, 70-71, 208-209, 224,
   356-364

Marriage and living arrangements, 25, 33, 36-38, 58-60,
   84, 89-90, 122, 131-165,
   169, 199-200, 202, 206-207,
   214, 218, 220-222, 246,
   284, 313, 347, 349

Mexican, 2-4, 6-13, 16-20, 22-
   27, 29-32, 36, 40-41, 43-46,
   48-52, 54-58, 60-61, 63, 65,
   67-68, 71-73, 75-82, 84-85,
   87-89, 91-101, 106-113, 115-
   121, 123-130, 132-133, 137-
   148, 150-156, 158-161, 164-
   165, 167, 172, 175, 177-178,
   181, 195-205, 210, 212-213,
   215-217, 222, 224, 225, 228,
   230, 232, 237, 249, 251,
   259, 266-273, 277-278, 280,
   285-286, 288-289, 291, 293-
   294, 297-298, 304-305, 312-
   313, 322-324, 329, 331, 333-
   336, 339-342, 344, 348-350,
   352, 355, 357, 362, 364

Migrant farm workers, 213,
   230

Migration (see Fertility,
general determinants of,
migration)

Minority group status (see
Fertility, general determinants of, minority group
status)

Peruvian, 91

Prenatal care, 170-178, 210,
   226, 234, 288

Puerto Rican, 6, 15, 23, 36-
   37, 52, 56, 58, 62, 66, 83,
   90-91, 104, 107, 113, 125,
   127, 135-136, 142-145, 148,
   157, 160, 170, 177, 179-180,
   184-191, 194, 202-204, 206,
   210, 212, 216-218, 222, 225,

Puerto Rican (cont'd)
   228, 234-235, 240, 248, 251,
   259, 268, 282, 287, 295-296,
   300-302, 308-309, 322-323,
   331, 339, 341-342, 344-345,
   347-352, 355-356, 360-361,
   363

Religion (see Fertility,
general determinants of,
religion)

Religiosity (see Attitudes,
religiosity)

Risk taking, 101, 174, 281

Sex education, 13, 27, 30, 51,
   68-71, 74-75, 105, 288, 357,
   359, 361

Sex roles (see Attitudes, sex
roles)

Sexual activity, 35, 55, 61,
   63, 68, 93, 113, 166-169,
   202, 209, 239, 241, 248,
   276, 279, 284, 313-314, 358,
   361-362

Sexually transmitted
   diseases, 167

Socioeconomic status (see
Fertility, determinants of,
socioeconomic status)

South American (see Central
and South American)

Sterility, 176

Sterilization, 27, 104, 175,
   224, 271, 284-285, 288-289,
   291-293, 295-304, 355

Urbanization, 24, 196

Utilization of services, 172,
   252, 258, 305, 353

About the Compiler

KATHERINE F. DARABI has lived and worked in Latin America and most recently has conducted research on adolescent pregnancy and childbearing in the United States. A faculty member at the Columbia University School of Public Health, she has contributed numerous articles to the *American Journal of Public Health, Community Development Journal, Studies in Family Planning,* the *Hispanic Journal of Behavioral Sciences, Obstetrics and Gynecology,* and *Adolescence.*